Obstetric Violence and the Birthing Body

Obstetric Violence and the Birthing Body: A Reading from Feminist Philosophy examines the phenomenon of violence against women and birthing subjects during medicalized birth from the viewpoint of diverse fields within feminist philosophy.

The phenomenon of obstetric violence—violence and the dehumanizing treatment of laboring women at the hands of medical staff—affects women and birthing persons all over the world, with dreadful consequences. This book argues that obstetric violence is a distinct form of violence against women that cannot be adequately understood simply by labeling it as "gender violence." It demonstrates how violent obstetric practices have been normalized and provides practical guidance for those seeking to influence social policies and create structural change within women's healthcare.

Obstetric Violence and the Birthing Body will be of use to women everywhere, health providers, policy makers, and students and researchers in many branches of feminist philosophy as well as other academic disciplines including public health, human rights, welfare, sociology, midwifery, medical anthropology, medical ethics, and law.

Sara Cohen Shabot is Associate Professor in the Philosophy Department and Chair of the Women's and Gender Studies Program at The University of Haifa, Israel, specializing in feminist philosophy, phenomenology, and philosophies of the body. Her present research and publications address feminist philosophical perspectives on childbirth and the maternal embodied subject.

Focus on Global Gender and Sexuality

A Feminist Approach to Sensitive Research
Designing the Clay Embodiment Research Method
Tricia Ong

Postfeminism, Postrace and Digital Politics in Asian American Food Blogs
Tisha Dejmanee

Israeli Masculinity, Sex Work, and Consumerism
Heteronormativity and Sexual Repertoires
Yeela Lahav-Raz

Reading Literature and Theory at the Intersections of Queer and Class
Class Notes and Queer-ies
Edited by Maria Olive Alexopoulos, Tomasz Basiuk, Susanne Hochreiter and Tijana Ristic Kern

Femicide in Latin America
A Growing Threat to Women's Security
Isabelle Vladoiu

Obstetric Violence and the Birthing Body
A Reading from Feminist Philosophy
Sara Cohen Shabot

For more information about this series, please visit: www.routledge.com/Focus-on-Global-Gender-and-Sexuality/book-series/FGGS

"This magnificent book demands that the reader rethink what birthing bodies and subjects are, and indeed what birth is. By exploring conceptions of birth as grotesque, erratic and uncertain it produces new insights into how birthing bodies are subjected to violence and shame. Brilliant, insightful and inspiring, this book speaks to the mind and the heart in finding new ways of restoring birthing to its rightful site as an act of awe."

Jonathan Herring, *Professor of Law, University of Oxford; DM Wolfe-Clarendon Fellow in Law, Exeter College, Oxford*

"Professor Cohen Shabot brings new depth of analysis to the universal experience of Obstetric Violence. Her powerful book outlines deeply held societal behavioral and existential conceptions of women and birthing persons that make violence against them normative. We can only change the structural violence of our societies through this understanding."

Annekathryn Goodman, *Professor of Obstetrics, Gynecology, Reproductive Biology, Harvard Medical School, Director Strength & Serenity MGH Global Initiative to End Gender-Based Violence*

"This book delivers a critical feminist intervention on obstetric violence. Sara Cohen Shabot's bold theoretical insight unsettles entrenched paradigms and illuminates birth as both a site of violence and horizon of possibility. A field-defining contribution that will resonate across disciplines."

Camilla Pickles, *Associate Professor of Biolaw, Durham University*

Obstetric Violence and the Birthing Body

A Reading from Feminist Philosophy

Sara Cohen Shabot

Routledge
Taylor & Francis Group
LONDON AND NEW YORK

First published 2026
by Routledge
4 Park Square, Milton Park, Abingdon, Oxon OX14 4RN

and by Routledge
605 Third Avenue, New York, NY 10158

Routledge is an imprint of the Taylor & Francis Group, an informa business

British Library Cataloguing-in-Publication Data
A catalogue record for this book is available from the British Library

ISBN: 978-1-032-96459-1 (hbk)
ISBN: 978-1-032-97457-6 (pbk)
ISBN: 978-1-003-59382-9 (ebk)

DOI: 10.4324/9781003593829

Typeset in Times New Roman
by Newgen Publishing UK

To my children, Noa and Eviatar, and my mother, Esther (*para ti, ma*)—with you three I have shared the pangs and joys of giving birth and being born, and of mothering and being mothered.

And to Ron—with you I share everything else, and, above all, love.

Contents

Preface

This book is the result of a decade's worth of work. I started writing about childbirth a few years after giving birth to my first child, Noa. When she was born, I was almost thirty-five years old: a fully adult woman and an academic with a PhD in philosophy. Nevertheless, birth caught me by surprise. My pregnancy was smooth and uneventful; I had time to digest the many changes that I was going through, mentally and physically. Birth, though, was something else. It was both the most extreme and wonder-provoking event I had ever experienced and, at the same time, an event in the face of which I felt helpless. I could not get a grip on birth. I tried, but everything seemed so blurry and so sharp at the same time, and I could not manage to understand this event during which unbearable pain had made my body burst and deliver my baby daughter to life outside of me. I experienced an epistemic crisis.

Almost immediately, I turned to philosophy to try to make sense of what had happened. I wrote a chapter on birth as both transcendence and immanence, as ambiguity, using Beauvoir, and then a paper on the special nature of childbirth pain (Cohen Shabot 2017b; Cohen Shabot 2017a). During that time, I also gave birth to my second child, Eviatar. This time, I hoped, birth would no longer be unfamiliar, but then it was: my son's birth turned out to be an experience that left me wounded, humiliated, broken. I felt lost. I had been robbed of my autonomy and treated as an object, with no care or compassion.

After I managed to pick up the pieces, I decided that I needed to continue researching and writing on the subject of childbirth, which, I had already discovered, was impressively under-researched in philosophy. Now, however, I knew that I had to focus on the violence

I had experienced during my second birth: my unexpectedly dreadful experience in a standard medical setting in a first-world country. I was truly surprised when my early investigations showed me that I was not alone—this was a global phenomenon that the literature (and, even earlier, activism) had already recognized as "obstetric violence." My first philosophical paper on the subject was dedicated to demonstrating that obstetric violence is not only medical violence but also a type of gender violence (Cohen Shabot 2016). Following that publication, a large corpus of research on obstetric violence as gender violence developed, including philosophical work by myself and others. In the present book, I offer the core philosophical reflections on obstetric violence that I have developed over the last decade.

This book sees light in the midst of a very difficult period for me, mainly on the personal front. These last years have been marked by chaos, illness, and painful losses within my family. Furthermore, since my own fiftieth birthday a few years ago, my already very present anguish over disease, debility, and death has only increased. And yet, researching and discussing birth feels to me like an oasis: a place where I can still reflect on and even celebrate life and creativity. Of course, this research is not particularly cheerful. Like many of my colleagues, I came to these subjects through trauma and loss. Yet I still find this field to be truly connected to life, love, care, and community, even when the research is about uncovering injustice and violence.

Above all, I keep looking at the experiences of pregnancy, birth, and motherhood with great philosophical perplexity and a strong sense of awe—as Dahan (2023) also puts it. For me personally, research on birth has been in great measure a sublimation, after many miscarriages, of my thwarted desire to experience one more birth—this one at home—and have a third child, as I so much wanted to. On the other hand, there is so much philosophical depth to this subject, so much to say about it from so many angles, that I often think that my personal history has actually just become an excuse to keep doing this research.

In truth, the work of all my dear colleagues in the field of birth studies inspires me and fills me with curiosity and excitement. For this, and for the fact that so many of you have also become a great source of support for me, both academic and otherwise, I am sincerely grateful. I never take this support for granted. Thus, I thank all my peers and friends who have accompanied me throughout this research and in my life over this last decade (and before that): my Beauvoirian colleagues, my colleagues in the Department of Philosophy at the University of Haifa, and especially my growing community of birth researchers and activists worldwide. You all know who you are.

I am grateful, as well, to my students in the Women's and Gender Studies Program at the University of Haifa, and to all who have listened to or read my work on birth and provided feedback—often bringing me to tears as you talked about how this work allowed you to finally make some sense of your own stories of trauma and violence.

For their kind support (not only financial) for the publication of this book, I deeply thank the Faculty of Humanities and the Research Authority at the University of Haifa. And, as always, I thank Marie Deer for her invaluable editorial suggestions and feedback.

My most important thanks go to Ron, my unconditional partner for more than twenty years now and the loving father of our children. Without Ron, none of this would be possible—not only because of his endless support, but because I would be a totally different person without him in my life. My gratitude also to Noa and Eviatar, who gave me the precious gift of birth and motherhood and have become my greatest inspiration, in general and for this book in particular. It is Ron, Noa, and Eviatar, finally, who bring me to writing, because day after day they ground me in life.

Acknowledgments of previous publications

Parts of this book were previously published in different forms, and I appreciate the permission to reprint them here.

Sections of the introduction and of Chapter One first appeared in "Making Loud Bodies 'Feminine': A Feminist-Phenomenological Analysis of Obstetric Violence" (2016), *Human Studies* 39 (2): 231–247, Springer Nature. Other parts of Chapter One were first published in "We Birth with Others: Towards a Beauvoirian Understanding of Obstetric Violence" (2021), *The European Journal of Women's Studies* 28 (2): 213–228.

Chapter Two is made up of reworked versions of "'Amigas, Sisters*: We Are Being Gaslighted*': Obstetric Violence and Epistemic Injustice" (2019), in *Childbirth, Vulnerability and Law: Exploring Issues of Violence and Control*, edited by Camilla Pickles and Jonathan Herring (Routledge), and "'You Are Not Qualified—Leave It to Us': Obstetric Violence as Testimonial Injustice" (2021), *Human Studies* 44 (4): 635–653, Springer Nature.

Lastly, parts of Chapter Three draw from "Unauthorized Intimate Examinations as/and Sexual Violence: Some Epistemic and Phenomenological Considerations" (2020), in *Women's Birthing Bodies and the Law: Unauthorized Intimate Examinations, Power and Vulnerability*, edited by Jonathan Herring and Camilla Pickles (Hart Publishing, an imprint of Bloomsbury Publishing Plc.), and "Why 'Normal' Feels So Bad: Violence and Vaginal Examinations during Labour—A (Feminist) Phenomenology" (2021), *Feminist Theory* 22 (3): 443–463.

All of these are reprinted with permission.

Introduction

The Problem of Obstetric Violence

In January of 2010, I gave birth to my younger son, knowing what I wanted from this birth and pretty convinced that this baby would be born the way I wanted. I went to the hospital in active labor, expecting the birth to go quickly, but things got messy: the baby would not descend, and my labor stopped. I was confined to my hospital bed, continuously monitored, and forbidden to move, waiting for hours in agonizing pain. My body—which I had experienced as strong and capable until I arrived at the hospital—became my enemy, feeling stiff, fragmented. As my labor went on, I was subjected to numerous medical interventions without my explicit consent, including a catheterization, the artificial rupture of my waters, and repeated painful vaginal examinations. I was told countless times that if labor did not progress quickly, they would need to perform a Caesarean section, otherwise my baby would die. I felt mute, deprived of agency.

Finally, my baby—large and healthy—was born vaginally. My perineum remained intact: no tearing, no need for stitches. This was a labor with apparently optimal results: no physical damage, healthy mother, healthy baby. Nothing to complain about; nothing to mourn. Nevertheless, that labor experience still haunts me and has informed almost all of my academic writing since that time. Today I can attest that I suffered from obstetric violence and that this was, in more ways than one, a traumatic experience.

I am not alone. I soon learned that the experience of traumatic birth as a consequence of violence in the labor room is pervasive, especially where childbirth is highly medicalized, almost exclusively controlled by medical authorities heavily influenced by capitalist and patriarchal values. Therefore, I offer here a feminist-philosophical analysis of the

DOI: 10.4324/9781003593829-1

widespread phenomenon of obstetric violence, to which thousands of parturient women[1] have fallen and continue to fall victim, sometimes with terrible consequences.[2]

Since I began writing on obstetric violence, a decade ago, the research has grown exponentially; hundreds of studies on the subject have been published. It has been analyzed from psychological, sociological, and anthropological perspectives and tackled by health researchers, law scholars, and scholars working in decolonial and postcolonial theories. An exhaustive review of these studies is beyond the scope of this book, but I will refer to a few of them, mainly those that provide compelling accounts of the latest literature and comprehensively analyze the subject of obstetric violence as discussed in a myriad of disciplines. Many more studies will be discussed or referred to in the following chapters.

Above all, I want to stress that the research on, and struggle against, obstetric violence began not in the Global North (where much of the recent literature on the subject has been produced) but rather in Latin America. For a comprehensive analysis of the Latin American struggle that gave birth to the concept of obstetric violence and initiated the protest against it through legislation and social activism see Sadler (2020; 2025.)

Some of the most thorough and illuminating recent studies on the multidisciplinary research into obstetric violence are those of Pickles (2023; 2024). Pickles exhaustively maps the history of the phenomenon and the concept, referring to studies within various disciplines and tracing the history of the struggle against obstetric violence and the development of the concept since its beginnings in Latin America, followed by extensive research and activism in the Global North. Pickles brings up this trajectory mainly in order to discuss the different terms that have been used to describe the phenomenon of violence against laboring women. She makes compelling arguments about two main aspects of the current conceptual discussion of obstetric violence. First, she makes it clear why the appropriate term for the phenomenon is, finally, "obstetric violence" (rather than other terms that have been used, including "mistreatment" and "abuse"). She rightly argues that "obstetric violence" best captures the structural dimensions of the phenomenon and also, crucially, respects the history behind the recognition of the phenomenon (beginning, as noted, with Latin American activism). She points out that the terms "mistreatment" and "disrespect and abuse" are preferred by healthcare professionals and institutions, who are the ones perpetrating this violence and thus should not have the right to name or define it. The term "mistreatment," in particular,

> hides the full extent of violence and abuse, ignores the broader context that drives violations during childbirth, and it undermines the development of comprehensive responses. It minimizes the central role of women as authoritative namers of their experiences through active discreditation of women's construction of violence and abuse. Further, it allows naming practices to be determined by the very individuals and institutions responsible for violence and abuse in childbirth. Consequently, the continued use of "mistreatment" merely expands and maintains the health professions' reach of power and control over all dimensions of childbirth, rather than challenge it.
>
> (Pickles 2023, 644)

Secondly, Pickles discusses the urgent issue of how exactly, and by whom, the boundaries of what does and does not constitute obstetric violence should be set. The recent exponential growth of discussions and research on obstetric violence has rendered this question urgently pressing, especially within law scholarship, which is demanding practical recommendations on how to approach the problem. "Everything Is Obstetric Violence Now" is part of the title of a recent article by Pickles, which, by presenting an exhaustive study of what has been considered to constitute obstetric violence, convincingly argues against defining obstetric violence too broadly, so that its true damage can be tackled in practice. Mainly, however, Pickles (2024) demonstrates that this limit-setting must be achieved through a meticulous investigation of the diverse violations constituting obstetric violence and concludes that, in order to know when we are seeing obstetric violence, we need to look for a "violation of physical and/or psychological integrity … occur[ring] in the context of labor and/or of childbirth, and [where] the subject of violence is the birthing woman, trans or non-binary person" (Pickles 2024, 644). This definition is both broad enough to allow new kinds of violations to be recognized as obstetric violence and limited enough to confine it to violence happening within the scene of labor and childbirth and affecting the laboring person themself.

In this book, as noted above, I offer an exclusively *feminist-philosophical* analysis, focusing on how obstetric violence is lived and experienced by birthing persons and why it is frequently described in terms not only of violence in general but of gender violence specifically: violence directed at women *because* they are women (or something other than cis-gender men).

Obstetric Violence

The phenomenon of obstetric violence, directly resulting from the pathologization and medicalization of labor, is thus recognized as structural violence—deriving from the very construction of medicalized birth (Bohren et al. 2015; Miller and Lalonde 2015). It has also been described as a clear form of gender violence (Herring 2019; Pickles 2019; Cohen Shabot 2016; Cohen Shabot and Korem 2018; Sadler et al. 2016), because the dehumanizing treatment that many birthing women undergo as part of hospitalized labor specifically targets them as women.

The confluence of structural and gender violence in the mistreatment, neglect, and abuse that women experience at the hands of medical staff during childbirth constitutes obstetric violence (Beck 2004a; Elmir et al. 2010; Harris and Ayers 2012; Simpson and Catling 2015; Thomson and Downe 2008). Obstetric violence includes verbal and physical violence that damages women emotionally, mentally, and physically, frequently to the point of trauma and partial or full PTSD (Beck 2004b; Beck and Casavant 2019). Obstetric violence—violence against women birthing in medicalized settings—is widely recognized as a structural phenomenon affecting innumerable women globally and systematically, a problem in urgent need of being solved (Bohren et al. 2015; Miller and Lalonde 2015; Sadler et al. 2016). Bohren et al. (2015), reviewing more than sixty studies from thirty-four countries, describe laboring women in medical facilities in different countries, across all socioeconomic levels, being exposed to disrespectful and abusive treatment. This includes physical violence and restraint (including tying a woman's legs to the gynecological table during a normal delivery; performing physical examinations without consent, previous personal introduction of the health professional, or explanation of the procedure; collective vaginal touches for technical education; digital cervical reduction; the use of Kristeller's technique to accelerate birth; routine amniotomy; and not allowing the patient to choose the best position for delivery); threats of violence towards the woman and her baby or of withholding medical care if she fails to follow staff orders; blaming the laboring woman for poor health outcomes for herself or her child; discrimination against poor women, immigrants, minorities, and women perceived as too young or too old; denial or lack of pain relief; and the performance of episiotomies, sutures, and invasive examinations without anesthesia. Researchers have identified seven types of mistreatment: *physical abuse; verbal abuse; sexual abuse; stigma and discrimination; failure to uphold medical standards of care; miscommunication between laboring women and medical staff;* and *issues resulting from the state of the healthcare system, including lack of resources and problematic policies.* It has been recognized as gender violence, not simply medical violence[3] (Cohen Shabot 2016; Cohen Shabot and Korem 2018; Sadler et al. 2016), and as being experienced very differently by white, Euro-American, middle-class women (like myself) than it is by marginalized, poor, or minority populations, a difference defined as "too much too soon" versus "too little too late" (Miller et al. 2016). (Research shows, however, that obstetric violence is also rampant in semi-developed countries, where childbirth has become more medicalized but a strong tradition of caring for human, especially women's, rights, is still largely missing (Béhague et al. 2002; Beken's 2001; Potter et al. 2001)). "Too much too soon" refers to medicalization and the overuse of technology in labor, which has been shown to diminish laboring women's self-image and sense of agency (Behruzi et al. 2013; Smeenk and ten Have 2003; Wolf 2012), while "too little too late" refers to a lack of technology and basic medical attention.[4] Racism and other forms of discrimination, too, have been shown to clearly affect and magnify obstetric violence (Altman et al. 2020; Chadwick 2019; Davis 2019). Davis (2019) delves into racism in medicalized childbirth, introducing the useful concept of "obstetric racism"—the structural racism at the core of medicalized childbirth that produces differential reproductive outcomes—demonstrating that neither "obstetric violence" nor "medical racism" alone can explain the increased harm done to nonwhite women in childbirth, regardless of their socioeconomic status.[5]

The phenomenon has been legally defined and penalized in some countries (Pérez D'Gregorio 2010) and recently recognized by the World Health Organization and the United Nations as an urgent global problem (Šimonović 2019; WHO 2018). There is now constant, copious research underway into the different forms that obstetric violence takes around the world and in different societies, as well as into its possible solutions (see for instance Perrotte et al. 2020 meta-review).

More and more studies are being done on the pervasiveness of obstetric practices that are not evidence-based, do not improve medical outcomes, and are performed on women in labor without their explicit consent, sometimes even in spite of their explicit refusal.[6] These studies demonstrate a clear relation between these interventions and the presence of post-traumatic stress disorder (PTSD) in new mothers. Fernández (2013) summarizes many of these studies, showing how traumatic births—as defined by mothers themselves—usually result from dehumanizing treatment of mothers by medical authorities,[7] often involving depriving laboring women of any agency. Women report feeling forced to undergo interventions without being truly informed about the processes and consequences; they feel disrespected and uncared for. The feeling of abuse these women report can be at least partially explained by the process of being transformed from a *Leib*, a living body infused with freedom and the possibility of transcendence, into a *Körper*, a passive body-object with no embodied agency and no possibility of active engagement with the world. Or, in Beauvoir's terms, being turned by the oppressor from an embodied ambiguous subject, immanent and transcendent at once, into pure immanence, pure facticity[8]:

> Words such as *barbaric*, *intrusive*, *horrific* and *degrading* were used by the women to describe the mistreatment they received from health care professionals … Other participants talked of feeling like a "lump of meat" or a "slab on a table" when describing the dehumanizing way in which they were treated during birth and described a total lack of acknowledgement of them as humans.
>
> (Fernández 2013, 48; emphasis in the original)

Wolf (2013) presents a compelling philosophical analysis of obstetric violence, describing medicalized childbirth as containing an implicit element of "metaphysical violence." Drawing on Žižek's (2008) analysis of the phenomenon of violence, Wolf claims that medicalized childbirth undermines a woman's very sense of self, her core being: it makes women into moral objects rather than subjects, canceling their epistemic authority, their embodied capabilities, and their sense of being a particular individual in labor (instead of just another woman in labor); the laboring woman herself does not even have to perceive it as violent for it to be recognizable as a clearly violent practice. Wolf compares a woman's situation in medicalized childbirth to that of alienated workers in capitalist societies:

> Returning to Žižek, the laborer who is a victim of objective, systemic violence under the everyday workings of capitalism often does not perceive the damage done. In fact, many actually willingly participate in the continuation of the capitalist, free market system that damages them. This is because the system works via practices that are deemed normal and natural—they are not violence, they are just the way things are. Similarly, women who experience metaphysical violence in childbirth may not perceive the damage done and may even support medicalized childbirth. This is not due to any deficiency or problem with the woman but rather results from the success that medicalized childbirth has had in establishing itself as the normal way of giving birth ... part of metaphysical violence in medicalized childbirth is the obfuscation of the problem—it works, in part, precisely by being able to function undetected under the guise of normal practice.
>
> (Wolf 2013, 109–110)

These analyses, however, ignore the genderedness of obstetric violence. We cannot properly explain the phenomenon without making sense of the dimension of gender (in addition to recognizing it as utterly dehumanizing and objectifying in general terms). Thus, I broaden the analysis of violent labor, showing how, if we want to grasp all its complexity and specificity, it must be understood not only as containing elements of dehumanization and objectification, in common with other forms of medicalization, but also in reference to its gendered aspects.[9]

In 2007, Venezuela was the first country to legally recognize the term *obstetric violence*,[10] thereby establishing a basis for acknowledging the violence done to women in childbirth as part of the more general, widespread violence of which women are victims in patriarchal societies. The Venezuelan law, included in the "Organic Law on the Right of Women to a Life Free of Violence," defines obstetric violence as

> the appropriation of the body and reproductive processes of women by health personnel, which is expressed as dehumanized treatment,

> an abuse of medication, and to convert the natural processes into pathological ones, bringing with it loss of autonomy and the ability to decide freely about their bodies and sexuality, negatively impacting the quality of life of women.
>
> (Pérez D'Gregorio 2010, 201)

The inclusion of terms and phrases such as "dehumanization," "abuse," "loss of autonomy," and "loss ... of women's ability to decide freely about their bodies and sexuality" suggests that this specific kind of violence can be best understood by appealing to analyses of gendered violence—and specifically sexual violence—and the objectification of women rather than through more general accounts of medical violence. This suggestion is strengthened by some women's use of the term *birth rape* to describe their experience of obstetric violence.

Birth Rape

Before discussing the idea of "birth rape" I want to add an important disclaimer: I do not argue that obstetric violence *is* rape. It is not necessary to equate the two ontologically nor to insist that every case of obstetric violence is rape to acknowledge the many reports from women (including women who have experienced previous sexual violence) who recognize their own experience of obstetric violence as "birth rape." A phenomenological analysis of these experiences is essential and could be highly productive in political and philosophical terms: The voices of women who experience their labor as a form of rape need to be heard and explored, though there is a tendency to want to silence them in an attempt to keep the category of rape untouched. I am aware that using the category of rape in this context might seem problematic, even scandalous, especially regarding its implications for the medical staff's intentions. But if we deal with these reports *phenomenologically* (thus avoiding any question of the staff's "real intentions"), we can listen to them and reflect on them without censuring them for using the term *rape*.

Several studies (Elmir et al. 2010; Fernández 2013; Kitzinger 2006) show parturient women using metaphors of rape to describe their experiences of obstetric violence. Rich (1986) and Martin (1987) write extensively and compellingly about the alienation from their body that numerous women report feeling after experiencing highly medicalized labors. Martin recounts many stories by women who felt almost annihilated, totally deprived of subjectivity, split from their bodies, and robbed while going through Caesarean sections, and in these stories she identifies the language of rape, quoting one woman saying: "It was like a feeling of rape, completely out of control. My body was totally violated. I felt nobody cared. You wear cheap clothes and a lot of makeup and if you're raped, it's your fault. I felt the same thing with the cesarean." Martin then quotes a study on Caesarean sections: "Women shudder at the memory of being tied on the table and completely vulnerable to a man wielding a knife" (Martin 1987, 84). In an autoethnographic study, the retired midwife and childbirth educator Shea Richland (2008) tells her own birth rape story: her first childbirth, at age seventeen, in 1969 America. What began as a normal birth became highly medicalized; she experienced tremendous fear and absolute loss of control while undergoing massive medical interventions undertaken with no explicit consent from her, denying her, among many other things, the possibility of even looking at her baby for hours after labor (completely sedated as she was). She only learned later that her baby had been pulled from her unconscious body with forceps, after she underwent an episiotomy that turned into a third-degree tear; her placenta was also removed manually by the doctor. Several years later, she had a vivid flashback to this during a conference on childbirth:

> I had, without warning, been taken back to the scene of a crime—a rape. My daughter's birth contained all the elements of a rape. I was taken to a strange place and told what to do. My clothes and personal possessions were taken from me. I was forced into an uncomfortable position and bound. I was threatened (it's hospital policy, don't make trouble). I was drugged and knocked unconscious. I was sexually assaulted: My vagina was cut and a man's tool (forceps) was inserted into my body. I was robbed. That which was most precious to me, my baby, was taken from me. All this was done against my will. Like most rape victims, I dried my tears, stuffed my pain and proceeded to get on with my life. Like many rape victims, I didn't report the crime nor did I seek help. I also didn't have a clue how profoundly or for how long these acts of violence would affect my life.
>
> (Martin 1987, 43)

Recent accounts of obstetric violence and birth rape demonstrate that this is not just something that happened fifty years ago: it is part of the current reality of medicalized childbirth. One case, a birth in California that was entirely caught on film by a family member, caused particular scandal. In its blog about violations of human rights in childbirth, the organization "Human Rights in Childbirth" documents the case as "Forced Episiotomy: Kelly's Story" (Hayes-Klein 2014). The story portrays a degree of obstetric violence similar to that in Richland's tale, but with the added circumstance that Kelly had already suffered from sexual violence before she underwent this violent childbirth; she had even informed the medical staff of that before putting herself in its hands. The document includes this description by the lawyer and birth-rights advocate Hermine Hayes-Klein:

> Another contraction comes. The nurse directs Kelly to pushpushpush gogogo. In the foreground, the doctor bustles with scissors and a medical cloth. He throws the cloth over Kelly's lower belly, exposing her perineum below it, and approaches with the scissors. Panting with the contraction, Kelly calls out desperately, "No, don't cut me!" … Kelly begs, "No! Why? Why can't we try?" The doctor's voice is authoritative now, even angry, as he responds: "What do you mean, 'Why?' That's my reason. Listen: I am the expert here." Kelly pleads, "But why can't I try?" The doctor answers, " 'Why can't I try?' You can go home and do it. You go to Kentucky."
>
> (Hayes-Klein 2014)

Many different forms of oppression and rights violations appear here, including the threat of physical violence (forced episiotomy), the appeal to authority as a legitimate reason for acting against the woman's will, and, finally, the attempt to belittle Kelly in "You go to Kentucky." (Kelly is not from Kentucky; Hayes-Klein points out that Kentucky here stands for "backwards" and "primitive" childbirth, mainly in the form of home birth.)

In Kelly's letter of complaint to the hospital after the birth, she describes the violations she experienced during her labor as birth rape:

> So then after he yelled at me he cut my Vagina twelve times. So before the episiotomy the nurse said it's only going to be a little cut. A little cut turned into Dr. A's horrific rage against me as a human

> being and against my will to begin with. I wanted to cry so badly and I was so horrified while he was cutting me. I could not believe after explaining I was raped twice that I was going to experience Birth Rape under your care.[11]
>
> (Hayes-Klein 2014)

These reports are an appalling testimony that women who undergo obstetric violence may suffer trauma much like that experienced by rape victims. Analyzing the phenomenology of rape, Lebowitz and Wigren (2005, 3) discuss some of the overwhelming themes that appear in rape victims' reports of their own subjective experience of the rape, including fear; helplessness; shame; loss of meaning and sustaining beliefs, legitimacy, and validation; self-blame and guilt; betrayal and loss of trust; isolation and alienation; a diminished sense of self; grief and loss; and anger and rage. These same themes pervade the accounts of women who experience obstetric violence, mainly those who describe their experience as equivalent to rape.

Why Is This Body Different from Other Bodies?

But why does obstetric violence feel like rape? And why do we feminize and sexualize the concept rather than simply talking about laboring women being turned into mechanical bodies, reduced to fleshed machines controlled and managed by medical authorities, pure vessels for a valuable product? What specifically characterizes the laboring body, making its objectification and belittlement different and more complex than for other kinds of bodies that medicine objectifies?

Writing almost thirty years ago, Leder (1998) explained the pervasive objectification of bodies in modern medicine, arguing that this kind of medicine adopts a model of the body drawn from Cartesian ideas of bodies as passive, marginal parts of mind-based selves. Dead bodies, Leder pointed out, are the bodies that medicine uses to learn about and find cures for living bodies' pathologies. It makes sense, then, that the best patient is the one that retains this passivity, this lack of movement or freedom, during the medical examination and/or intervention:

> The epistemological primacy of the corpse has shaped … medical technology, … training and practice. Medical education still begins with the dissection of a cadaver, just as the clinical case ends in the

> pathologist's lab. In between, the living patient is often treated in a cadaverous or machine-like fashion. We see this, for example, in the traditional physical examination. The patient is asked to assume a corpse-like pose, flat, passive, naked, mute. The entire ritual and context serves to reduce the living body to something almost dead. Personal identity is stripped away as the patient is removed from his or her habitual surroundings, activities, even clothes. Then, too, the patient's voice is, for long stretches, silenced.
>
> (Leder 1998, 121)

Laboring women express their objectification by medical authorities similarly (Martin 1987, 54–67; Wolf 2013, 105–109). This becomes especially clear in the feelings of anger and impotence women report when they are "comforted" after a traumatic birth with the phrase: "at least you have a healthy baby." Women hear this over and over, reinforcing their feeling of being pure flesh, a body-machine in the service of a higher end, a (now empty) vessel (Martin 1987, 65). But obstetric violence is more than just the usual objectification by doctors who want their patients to lie passive on the examination table. This difference derives mainly from the laboring body's profound erotic charge and remarkable strength, both of which need to be tamed by patriarchal powers. This is an active body, paradigmatic of the body as "I can"; a productive body, whose product is highly valuable to society; and a highly sexual body. As a feminine body, though, which is not supposed to have such features, it "demands" to be subjugated. At the same time, it is a vulnerable body, making it particularly open to violation and exploitation.

Women in labor perform an extremely difficult, physically consuming, sometimes excruciatingly painful task. Childbirth need not be essentialized—made sublime, beautiful, "natural"—for us to recognize its powerful, active character. Labor is totally incongruent with the myth of delicate, weak femininity. The laboring body is thus almost an oxymoron: the "feminine body" in the highest sense (birthing, accomplishing the task of femininity, revealing the "mysterious essence" of women), but also a strong, active, creative body, capable of enduring and recovering from the splitting of its flesh. This makes it dangerous, prone to domestication and control.

Childbirth also has a deeply sexual dimension that the medicalized model almost completely erases: childbirth results from pregnancy, itself almost always a product of sex. Moreover, except in Caesarean sections,[12] childbirth involves our genitals. A key principle in midwifery is that the more the labor is allowed to embrace its sexual aspects, the better it progresses. Ina May Gaskin, an American midwife and midwifery theoretician, writes: "sex is *the* central fact of reproductive behavior from conception to birth" (Gaskin 2003, 239; emphasis in the original). It seems plausible that women's description of obstetric violence as rape is connected to the perception of labor and birth as sexual.

In the next chapter, I present a more fully fleshed phenomenological analysis of the motives for the restraint of women in labor through violence, illuminating and understanding them precisely as originating in the patriarchal command to domesticate and silence women's bodies and sexualities. I also use phenomenology to demonstrate the primary damage that obstetric violence inflicts on laboring persons as being not loss of autonomy but rather loss of connection, of *being-with-others*, being supported and held—which is critical for constructing and sustaining subjectivity and thus, also, for a positive, non-alienated, non-traumatic birthing experience.

Notes

1 I use "birthing women," "birthing persons," and "birthing subjects" interchangeably since obstetric violence is a form of gender violence, directed not only toward women but also toward gender minorities giving birth who do not self-define as women. But we must also recognize that the great majority of birthing subjects are still women; thus, the phenomenon of obstetric violence should be understood primarily as one of violence against women.

2 As I note later, I deal with the phenomenon of obstetric violence mainly as experienced by white, Western, middle-class women, who are, in general, more exposed to medicalization and technology in labor. In feminist terms, the history of medicalized childbirth is interestingly complex: attempts to find medical relief from childbirth pain originated in desperate calls from women and feminist opposition to the suffering of childbirth that it had frequently been considered, throughout history, "natural" and "moral" for women to undergo. For countless women who decide to challenge this "natural destiny," numbing labor pain remains an empowering act (Baker 2010; Smeenk and ten Have 2003; Wolf 2012). Nevertheless, as childbirth became increasingly medicalized, many women felt disempowered by the very technologization of labor. Extreme numbing practices (like the "twilight sleep" used in America from the 1950s through the 1970s, rendering birthing women almost completely unconscious) became common,

diminishing laboring women's self-image and sense of control or agency (Behruzi et al. 2013; Smeenk and ten Have 2003; Wolf 2012).

3 This book deals exclusively with obstetric violence in medicalized settings. Women also experience mistreatment, even trauma, in midwife-led births outside medicalized settings—as in home births (Baker 2010; Charles 2013). However, violence experienced in these contexts is not recognized as "obstetric violence" in the research and is beyond the scope of this book.

4 Initially, this distinction was thought to characterize the differences between affluent and low-to-middle-income countries. Miller et al. (2016), however, propose that the two extremes coexist globally because of social and health inequities within countries. Thus, they argue, "a global approach to quality and equitable maternal health, supporting the implementation of respectful, evidence-based care for all, is urgently needed" (2176).

5 The case of Serena Williams—who suffered from obstetric violence mainly in the form of testimonial injustice done to her by the medical staff during her childbirth—is enlightening. This was a clear case of "obstetric racism," because Williams's wealth and prestige did not shield her from this damage. Dawes Gay (2018) reports:

> "When discussing Williams's maternal-health emergency, it's vital to address the role played by racism and racial discrimination—a requirement to sustainably address the United States' growing maternal-health problem. Black women are nearly four times more likely to die from pregnancy and childbirth than white women, and are also more likely to experience a severe maternal morbidity such as a heart attack, hemorrhage, sepsis, or blood clots like Williams did, regardless of their level of education or income. In fact, data from the New York City Department of Health show that black college-educated women were more likely than white women who hadn't completed high school to experience adverse maternal-health outcomes. Knowledge and money aren't enough to save black women, because racism trumps all."

6 Women can also be disempowered within the nonmedicalized, midwifery model of childbirth, even though that disempowerment may not result from violence. Charles (2013) reflects on the deep feelings of incompetence, frustration, and shame many women experience after "failing" to give birth without medical intervention; for some women, the "midwifery model" may be as disappointing as the medicalized one (see also Baker 2010). I do not analyze this kind of disempowerment here. In addition, I do not deal with the consequences of obstetric violence for the babies being born. Studies show benefits for babies delivered in a quiet environment and allowed to spend the first hours of life close to their mothers and undisturbed (Bodner et al. 2011; Salgado et al. 2013; Vieira et al. 2010; Wagner 2001). However, since these studies also, and mainly, show that

babies benefit in the long run from "good attachment," which mostly has to do with how the main caregiver interacts with the baby, the benefit to a baby of having a satisfied mother (whether or not her labor was medicalized) may be the key here.

7 It might be argued that because this is not perceived as violence by the obstetricians (who may consider it doing their best for the woman and baby), we cannot call it violence, since violence must be intentional to be counted as such. Landau (2010, 70), for instance, argues that explicit intention is a constitutive element of violence. Without attempting any philosophical reflection here on the ontological possibility of unintended violence, it is mandatory to stress that the concept of (intentional or unintentional) obstetric violence has been recognized by law and, more importantly, experienced and reported as such by a great number of women. However, Wolf's (2013) illuminating analysis of medicalized childbirth as essentially violent, from which I quote later on, is based on Žižek's (2008) concept of metaphysical violence, contending that violence must be intentional to be considered real violence.

8 This is precisely how the oppression of women has functioned, per Beauvoir: men have projected immanence onto women, falsely believing that they (men) are absolute transcendence while women are absolute Others, pure immanence, pure flesh. Men project their abject parts onto women and consequently deprive themselves of freedom, wrongly believing that they themselves are absolute freedom. By forbidding women to enter the dialectical subject-to-subject process, men deny themselves, paradoxically, their own freedom. By reducing women to their bodies, to pure immanence, pure facticity, while considering themselves as constituted by pure transcendence, a distilled freedom that is not mingled with embodiment nor intertwined with flesh, men also deny women the possibility of developing themselves as moral subjects with moral freedom. See Scarth (2004, 99–121) and Arp (2001, 138–40).

9 The assertion that obstetric violence is a form of gender violence and must be understood as structural rather than behavioral violence is central to my argument. This means that the medical staff is not necessarily aware of performing this kind of violence, often unconsciously perpetrating an existing violent structure (or, in some cases, attempting to resist that structure). In her compelling study of obstetric violence in Spain, Bellón Sánchez (2014, 27–29) uses Foucault's (2003) concepts of "biopower" and "authoritative knowledge" to situate the phenomenon of obstetric violence within the wider phenomenon of medical violence resulting from medicine's excessive power over bodies in contemporary Western societies and from the unquestioned authority that medical workers have been given. This wider phenomenon of medical violence, however, is also clearly gendered: Bellón Sánchez shows that women, and especially their reproductive processes,

have been particularly vulnerable to it. Modern medicine—deeply androcentric from its beginnings and to this day—endorses and reproduces male values and is particularly concerned with controlling female bodies (especially their reproductive processes and sexuality) while safeguarding male hegemony, as many feminist critiques of medicine argue. Obstetrics, with its intimate relation with human reproduction and female sexuality, Bellón Sánchez asserts, is especially prone to chauvinism and controlling practices (Bellón Sánchez 2014, 37). She discusses obstetric violence as another facet of the strict control exercised over women's bodies through "biopower" and medical "authoritative knowledge": women, barely considered to be "epistemic agents," have been largely excluded from the production of medical knowledge, including obstetrics. These systems of knowledge construe women as passive objects awaiting instructions regarding their condition (healthy/unhealthy or able/unable). Bellón Sánchez reviews literature showing many birthing women who do not trust their bodily experiences until the doctor confirms them as "real," and several cases in which the consent of the doctor and the medical staff—not of the woman—is needed for the delivery to "officially" start or for the woman to begin pushing (Bellón Sánchez 2014, 30). Medical violence towards women, and obstetric violence in particular, must be recognized as part of more general pervasive violence towards women. Obstetric violence may be seen as a consequence of both the excessive power of hegemonic, androcentric medical authority and the ubiquity of violence against women.

10 Argentina and Mexico followed (in 2009 and 2014, respectively). The term was introduced in Venezuela following social campaigns during the 1980s to improve sexual health and reproductive rights; the actual legal phrase "obstetric violence" was used for the first time in the 2007 document, as one of nineteen different types of punishable violence against women (Bellón Sánchez 2014, 54). Bellón Sánchez suggests (50–62) that the coinage of this term in developing Latin American countries probably had to do with the omnipresence there of chauvinism and the resulting violations of women's rights, along with a greater awareness of and willingness to contend with that sexism and gender inequality in those societies in recent decades. For a comprehensive discussion of the Latin American struggle and activism against obstetric violence, see Sadler (2020; 2025).

11 See Reed (2008) for another very disturbing report of birth rape.

12 Note, however, that even emergency Caesarean sections involving no genital manipulation are also frequently reported by women as rape. Childbirth appears to have a sexual dimension even when it becomes a Caesarean section; the feeling of being tamed, sometimes almost coerced, into the procedure and of being cut by the doctor's knife might be enough to make women feel raped. This complicates the assumption that the involvement of genitals and genital manipulations are the main reason these coerced births are perceived as rape.

1 The Phenomenological Perspective

Silenced Bodies, Solitary Bodies

Obstetric violence appears to be a complex, multilayer phenomenon. On the one hand, it has much in common with the more general experience of alienation and objectification within medicalization. The dehumanization some victims of obstetric violence experience matches the feeling that patients report in a variety of other dehumanizing medical scenarios: being turned into a passive object, a piece of flesh, without agency. On the other hand, obstetric violence appears to be unique in being directed almost exclusively at women and experienced mostly as gender violence, an affront to and banishment of their otherwise healthy, powerful, sexual, and creative embodied subjectivities.

This is why an analysis using feminist phenomenology—as "gendered phenomenology or a phenomenology of gender and gendered experience" (Fisher 2000, 37)—will be helpful for understanding and thematizing the complex, unique, and deeply gendered character of obstetric violence.

"Throwing Like a Girl," or the Domestication of Women's (Laboring) Bodies

Focusing on purposeful embodied activities in general and, specifically, the activity of throwing a ball, Young (1980) offers a careful, compelling explanation of why feminine bodies, from a very young age, behave differently from masculine bodies. Her core argument is that the important differences between men's and women's motility, starting in early childhood, are not determined by biology but result from how gendered cultural and social expectations affect people's core selves, to the point that both women and men incorporate and

DOI: 10.4324/9781003593829-2

recognize these differences as if they were the product of an unchangeable nature. In patriarchal and sexist societies, she reports, men are much more able to use their own bodies integrally, relating to them as a capable and forceful tool for self-expression and the accomplishment of teleological activities, while women are much more alienated from their bodies and their strength. Women approach activities hesitantly, with inherent insecurity: they perceive their own bodies as essentially feeble, incapable, and constantly requiring support and protection. Women are expected to keep their bodies as closed as possible: they are always vulnerable to attack or penetration. Young (1980) claims that if our possibilities in the world "depend on the mode and limits of the bodily 'I can'" (per Merleau-Ponty 1995 [1945]), then feminine existence is constructed as a perpetual "I cannot" (Young 1980, 146).

Young describes the tension women experience when they are directed, taught, or expected to domesticate their motile and creative bodies. Recalling Beauvoir, she argues that men are not usually split from their bodies: they are free to use them, to move, extend, and reach through them. They are one with their bodies, commonly at home in them. But women are alienated from their bodies: expected not to work through them, achieve things with them, or expand or gain power through them. Women's bodies are not supposed to express their capabilities:

> We often experience our bodies as a fragile encumbrance, rather than the media for the enactment of our aims. We feel as though we must have our attention directed upon our body to make sure it is doing what we wish to do, rather than paying attention to what we want to do *through* our bodies … We have more of a tendency than men to greatly underestimate our bodily capacity.
>
> (Young 1980, 144; emphasis in the original)

Women almost never accept this attitude towards their bodies, however, without a sense of conflict. Women experience themselves as "*inhibited intentionalit[ies]*" (Young 1980, 146; emphasis in the original), both projecting themselves towards goals and failing to reach them because of the overwhelming feeling that their bodies lack strength, capability. This inner contradiction arises from the gap, the space for resistance, that always remains within the subject: even when the dominant gaze has almost completely objectified it, the subject keeps reaching for transcendence. Thus, the paradoxes of feminine existence

> have their root in the fact that feminine existence does not experience the body as a mere thing—a fragile thing, which must be picked up and coaxed into movement, a thing which exists as *looked at and acted upon* … The objectified bodily existence accounts for the self-consciousness of the feminine relation to her body and resulting distance she takes from her body. As human, she is a transcendence and subjectivity, and cannot live herself as mere bodily object. Thus, to the degree that she does live herself as mere body, she cannot be in unity with herself, but must take a distance from and exist in discontinuity with her body.
>
> (Young 1980,148, 154; emphasis in the original)

The "essence" of feminine existence in patriarchal, sexist societies is to be objectified (Young draws here again on Beauvoir). Women always face a lose/lose situation: if they embrace and internalize their objectification, they experience themselves as split from their bodies, alienated from their embodied existence. But if they resist objectification, they also lose femininity and are usually either marginalized and despised or else immediately (often violently) put in their place:

> The objectifying regard which "keeps her in her place" can also account for the spatial modality of being positioned and for why women frequently tend not to move openly, keeping their limbs enclosed around themselves. To open her body in free active and open extension and bold outward directedness is for a woman to invite objectification.
>
> (Young 1980,154)

Returning to the laboring body and the violence performed on it, and to the difference between this violence and objectification and that performed in other medical scenarios, I propose that the active, creative, powerful, open body in labor, which is not shy or weak but at its core loud and almost irreverent, is precisely the "anti-feminine" body that has to be "put in its place," the threatening body that requires domestication by medical authorities. The violence performed against the birthing body does not just express the general control and objectification characteristic of medical scenarios but is specifically an action against a subversive, rebelling femininity, one that contests alienation, attempting to be one with its body, to feel at home within its embodied existence. Women in labor frequently come to recognize themselves as subjects, as enabled, unalienated embodied subjectivities: they enact a repudiation of their condition as objects and show a striking tendency to become authentic ambiguous subjects. The laboring process is one of the few opportunities for women to experience a situation of subjectivity through embodiment, in which they are not alienated from their bodies but deeply identified with them: in Beauvoir's terms, ambiguously conjoining transcendence with immanence.[1]

Countless labor stories (Gaskin 2003; Gaskin 2011; Powers 2009) describe labor as an integrative experience, compounding a strong sense of raw, uncontrollable embodiment with a clear sense of agency and self-sufficiency. Lundgren's phenomenologically informed study of the "meaning of giving birth" (2011) includes multiple reports reflecting this position, what Lundgren calls "women being subjects" in the process of labor:

> Well, it was so powerful. It was unlike anything else. As in very bad weather, such as a very heavy thunderstorm, a snowstorm or something. You can't control it. Something was happening regardless of what you do. I must say it's very, very groovy.
>
> (Lundgren 2011)

And from another report:

> You get concentrated when the pain comes and feel that the pain is developing something … to follow and see the connection in relation to the opening. During my last delivery, it was more like … no I don't want this. But now I was no longer a victim. Instead, I was more in control of myself, you may say.
>
> (Lundgren 2011, 122–123, quoted reports)

Laboring bodies are violently turned into objects not only because this is comfortable for the medical staff—passive Cartesian corpses being easier to handle than live bodies with desires and particularities—but mainly because they are feminine bodies threatening their own passive femininity: bodies acting from immanence, reaching towards transcendence; living, vigorous, sexual bodies challenging patriarchy. Their sexuality appears to be not commodified but self-owned: in charge of itself, not existing purely as object-for-the-other. This body, therefore, has to be put in its place, reminded again and again of its "inherent passivity." The sick feminine body might even receive more tolerance from the system than the well one: if you are weak and in need of help, you are feminine and will be helped, but if you threaten to erode the essence of femininity with your noisy, exuberant body, you will be domesticated and violently put in your place.

Rape is the ultimate tool for putting women in their place. It reminds women of their inherent condition in patriarchy, as objects to be owned instead of subjects to interact with. Young speaks about this as well:

> The threat of being seen is, however, not the only threat of objectification which the woman lives. She also lives the threat of invasion of her body space. The most extreme form of such spatial and bodily invasion is the threat of rape … I would suggest that the enclosed space which has been described as a modality of feminine spatiality is in part a defense against such invasion … The woman lives her space as confined and enclosed around her at least in part as projecting some small area in which she can exist as a free subject.
>
> (Young 1980, 154)

In labor, the very small area in which women can otherwise exist as free subjects threatens to become meaningfully extended. Through the extreme implement of birth rape, this space is coercively reduced back to its "proper" size. This is not to imply that the medical staff is necessarily conscious of participating in this reproduction and perpetuation of patriarchal violence. They could even be seen as victims of patriarchal values themselves.

Reconceiving Obstetric Violence: When Integrity and Independence Are Not Enough

Obstetric violence, however, reduces women's subjectivity in labor not only by denying women control, independent decisions, and embodied integrity but also, significantly, by damaging the social, communal character of childbirth. Obstetric violence has frequently been understood as impeding autonomy in the traditional sense: preventing individual decision-making, agency, and control over the body[2] (Baker et al. 2005; Pickles 2015; Pickles 2019; Smeenk and ten Have 2003; Vedam et al. 2017; Wagner 2001; Wolf 2012[3]). I argue, however, that obstetric violence—necessarily involving the presence of others—happens to a woman in a specific state of embodied vulnerability and can destroy subjectivity by failing to recognize that vulnerability, banning support and demolishing relationships and interdependence between laboring women and their significant others during childbirth. This argument introduces a conceptual shift, reframing the phenomenon as a moment where vulnerability is misrecognized and it is ambiguity, relationships, and support (rather than autonomy in the traditional sense) that are obstructed. This violence can now be recognized as cutting the links to our bodies and the world (otherwise accentuated during childbirth) that constitute our phenomenological condition, not merely hurting the "autonomous subject."[4]

Thus, in obstetric violence, the social quality of birth is shredded and obfuscated, forbidding interpersonal relations based on recognition and solidarity while exploiting the laboring woman's vulnerability, and frequently giving her patronizing protection rather than care and embodied connection. Beauvoir's idea of the authentic embodied subject as necessarily *ambiguous*—simultaneously immanent and transcendent, inescapably linked to the world and its others—is useful here for constructing a new understanding of how obstetric violence happens and what constitutes its damage.

Using Beauvoir's (1948; 2011) ideas of the situated and relational subject (along with Butler's [2016] idea of vulnerability, which has much in common with Beauvoir's conceptualizations), I present a more productive idea of obstetric violence: as violence that prevents ambiguity, impeding connection and interdependence rather than only, or mainly, hindering bodily integrity and self-determination.

More recent accounts of this subject as constructed of, and always dependent on, relations have also been proposed, as an alternative to versions of the self emphasizing individual autonomy and independence. Herring, for instance, offers a rich and compelling study of the relational self (versus the individual self) and the resulting concept of "relational autonomy"—challenging the "traditional conception of autonomy" (Herring 2020, 16). Herring argues for this much more complex and multilayer view of the self and its autonomy as a needed critique of the patriarchal liberal conception of the subject—a critique that might produce more accurate, productive understandings in legal contexts as well. His "relational autonomy" is an autonomy "not based on the concepts of free will and self-sufficiency":

> The ideal of relational autonomy is not the self-contained, independent, rational being. Rather, true autonomy is found within relationships. Where our decisions are made with and supported by others. Where our goals are mixed up with the decisions of others. The ideal autonomous person is not the lone businessman striving off to work protected by his suit and briefcase, but the mother changing the nappy.
>
> (Herring 2020, 18)

Feminist accounts, however, especially Beauvoir's, still provide the basis for these new conceptions of autonomy (as Herring (2020, 7) himself recognized), and they are most illuminating when they expose how profoundly their critiques are rooted within embodied experience. Thus, I focus here on how, using Beauvoir's pivotal conception of the ambiguous, embodied subject as constructed through others and Butler's idea of ontological corporeal vulnerability deriving from that, we might create new, more precise ways to understand the damage done by obstetric violence.

As already noted, obstetric violence has so far been recognized mainly as impeding laboring women's bodily autonomy and freedom of choice. Neoliberal concepts of the "ideal subject" as sovereign and independent dominate much of the discourse on obstetric violence and its damage; using the language of traditional autonomy, "freedom," and "independence," they frequently claim that what is lost is a subject who was complete, independent, and enclosed before the violent event but is damaged and broken by the system.

I do not claim that what is lost in obstetric violence is unrelated to loss of the power to decide freely how our specific, personal labor will develop. Disregard for birth plans and women's expressed preferences and decisions is typical of descriptions of the phenomenon (Baker et al. 2005). Nevertheless, the neoliberal patriarchal account of subjectivity and autonomy is not the best suited to describing the evil of obstetric violence; rather, it is the feminist (and especially feminist-phenomenological) account of subjectivity, conceived as inherently dependent, relational, ambiguously linked with the world and others, and essentially embodied and vulnerable (and the account of autonomy constructed in its image), that offers the best explanatory power for obstetric violence's wrongdoing. Moreover, what usually undergirds narratives of loss of agency after traumatic or violent births is the feeling of loneliness and detachment resulting from the lack of recognition, by the staff or others present at the labor, of the laboring woman's always-already situated and relational subjectivity, which is all the more present, in her state of heightened vulnerability and openness, during childbirth.

Below, I relate some examples that show a central characteristic of obstetric violence as consisting in its victim being unseen, losing a corporeal link with the world, being denied recognition of her inherent vulnerable condition. I then show how Beauvoir's "ambiguity" and Butler's "vulnerability" can help us make sense of these experiences.

The Violent Birth as a Solitary Birth[5]

In a meta-ethnography of women's perceptions and experiences of traumatic birth,[6] Elmir et al. (2010) show that a crucial factor of a traumatic birth is the birthing woman feeling "invisible or out of control." It is interesting to note that in several papers on obstetric violence, researchers describe this out-of-control feeling as mainly involving laboring women feeling alone or abandoned, being disregarded, excluded from decisions being made by medical staff about the progress of their own labor, rather than the women feeling that they could not control their bodies, that their bodies were behaving unexpectedly or in a strange or untrustworthy way or because of excessive pain or any particular obstetric intervention:

> Researchers reported that women's opinions were ignored … Information from healthcare professionals was not forthcoming, and women felt as though these people were "faceless" … or invisible … They felt betrayed … *Women believed that the lack of control and involvement in decision-making was primarily due to the fragmented care and lack of continuity in care, resulting in disconnections and lack of knowledge.*
>
> (Elmir et al. 2010, 2145, 2147; emphasis added)

This "fragmented care" results in inhumane treatment: women are turned into objects, rather than subjects to be cared for. Countless reports cite this inhumanity as a central feature of traumatic birth and obstetric violence: women report having felt fragmented in their bodies, like failing machines in for repairs, sometimes manipulated like pieces of meat, with no agency whatsoever, exposed to the gaze of strangers without being asked, and transparent, as though they did not exist as subjects, as though they were just data (Beck 2004a; Beck 2004b; Elmir et al. 2010; Martin 1987; Thomson and Downe 2008). A recent study of childbirth trauma in Irish first-time mothers (Byrne et al. 2017) clearly shows isolation, infantilization, and disregard by the staff to be central features of perceived violence in childbirth, leading to trauma:

> In failing to attain information or to achieve collaboration during childbirth, these women felt undermined and excluded. The failure to acknowledge the mother within childbirth as an informed individual or to include her in the experience through the sharing of information, may have facilitated the development of trauma for these women in creating a sense of exclusion and isolation as Cora stated, *Sort of feeling cut off was part of the trauma.*
>
> (Byrne et al. 2017, 5; emphasis in the original)

Byrne et al. also report these women feeling "dismissed, dehumanised and passive," as though they had been "acted upon" rather than being active actors in their labors (Byrne et al. 2017, 5). Women feel that their bodies are invaded, violated; they describe experiences of detachment and dissociation while enduring the violent birth. Above all, this study shows how "*a non-collaborative childbirth may facilitate the development of birth trauma*" (Byrne et al. 2017, 8; emphasis mine); it speaks, once again, of the critical importance of communication, caring, and the birthing woman feeling that she is "someone" in labor, rather than "something," only the carrier of the coming baby. In the words of one of the study's participants: "What about me? I'm still … I'm not just an incubator like (Rebecca)" (Byrne et al. 2017, 5).

After violent births, women report feeling trapped, anxiously confined in the traumatic experience, unable to transcend it; they also feel depressed, angry, sometimes suicidal. Women's capacity for intimacy, for intimate touch with both their baby and their partner, is severely affected after traumatic labors, as is their sexuality (Ayers et al. 2006; Elmir et al. 2010).

Harris and Ayers show that the most significant elements of a traumatic birth relate to the flawed interpersonal relationships developed between laboring women and staff. Women report the experience of being ignored as a core interpersonal cause of birth trauma, followed by lack of support, poor communication, being abandoned, and being put under pressure (Harris and Ayers 2012,1170). Feeling unassisted, unsupported, uncared for—deprived of a subjectivity that is truly sustained and contained by others—these are clear characteristics of violent and traumatic births. Studies of obstetric violence and traumatic birth conclude that support, caring, respect for women's choices, and an overall improvement in communication between women and medical staff are mandatory steps in any attempt to avoid such negative experiences (Byrne et al. 2017; Elmir et al. 2010; Harris and Ayers 2012; Simpson and Catling 2015).

Beauvoir's Situated and Ambiguous Subject

Beauvoir's idea of the ambiguous, situated subject can help us understand and formulate what precisely is lost when laboring women undergo obstetric violence. Beauvoir's phenomenological conceptualization of the subject—developed in her early ethical works such as *Pyrrhus and Cinéas* (2004 [1944]) and *The Ethics of Ambiguity* (1948 [1947]) and later on in *The Second Sex* (2011 [1949])—is the opposite of the Cartesian one: Beauvoir's subject is never alone, never constructed in isolation, nor is it purely mental; indeed, it is deeply embodied. Beauvoir's carnal subject is always open to and dependent on its others. It is always the other who can provide me with real, moral freedom, as it is the other who might steal this freedom from me: "only man can be an enemy for man; only he can rob him of the meaning of his acts and his life because it also belongs only to him alone to confirm it in its existence, to recognize it in actual fact as freedom" (Beauvoir 1948, 82). Thus, it is the other who gives meaning to my acts and projects, recognizing them and interpreting them. I need the other to be free so that I myself can be recognized as freedom: "We need others in order for our existence to become founded and necessary" (Beauvoir 2004, 129). The ethical choice constitutes the only possible authentic choice: if I desire to have my own subjectivity truly recognized and valued, I need free others who can give meaning to my projects. "To will oneself free is also to will others free" (Beauvoir 1948, 73).[7]

Beauvoir's subject is ambiguous in that it is always situated, particularly embodied, located in a concrete time and place, and thus *singularly* itself—but also always carnally open and reaching out, and thus more than (only) itself:

> It is because my subjectivity is not inertia, folding in upon itself, separation, but, on the contrary, movement toward the other that the difference between me and the other is abolished, and I can call the other mine. Only I can create the tie that unites me to the other, I create it from the fact that I am not a thing, but a project of self toward the other, a transcendence.
>
> (Beauvoir 2004, 93)

Ambiguity thus points to how we are simultaneously individuals and entwined with others: for Beauvoir, writes Kruks: "the lived body is the interface between self and world and so also between self and others" (Kruks 2012, 36). The lived body is ambiguously immanent and transcendent, facticity surpassed by projects. In the world but *not* the world, it is essentially connected to others although never completely lost or absorbed in the other (Beauvoir 1948, 12–13).[8]

Analyzing Beauvoir's ambiguity and its expression within her existentialist ethics, Keltner further points to the complexity of conceiving the subject as both separated from and intimately linked to its others:

> Contra the trend of critique against existentialism as solipsistic, Beauvoir insists that the ethics that existentialism proposes is the only ethics that can account for a philosophy of existence that insists simultaneously on the social bond as equally primordial to the separation of the existent … Beauvoir seeks an account of the ambiguous phenomenon not just of subjectivity as an active existent between transcendence and immanence, but also of the ambiguity of the "indissoluble" "me-others" relation (*EA*, 72; *PC*, 104) through an account of separation and connection.
>
> (Keltner 2006, 205–206)

Thus, Beauvoir's subjectivity cannot be exhausted by a neoliberal idea of subjectivity as (even potentially) absolutely independent and sovereign. This emphasis on the subject's ineluctable existence with others and not as an atomistic, individual self is also evident in how Beauvoir's ideas appear to be nourished by the Heideggerian *Mitsein* and the Merleau-Pontian conception of subjectivity as always already situated and carnally intertwined with the world and with others.[9]

Beauvoir's *Mitsein*, though, does not at all foresee a harmonious existence.[10] Being ambiguously tied to the world and to others—never alone, self-contained, or completely independent—means that separation and difference are necessarily sought within a world of shared meanings and thus, frequently, through conflict:

> For Beauvoir, humans are *Mitsein*, but this *Mitsein* can be lived either in separation and conflict or in friendship and solidarity. *Mitsein*, for her, then, does not mean that humanity is one and that everyone has the same goals and aspirations, living in some kind of friendly symbiosis. *Mitsein* is not an ethical concept, nor is it connected to authenticity. It expresses simply the fact that human reality is a being-with.
>
> (Gothlin 2003, 58)

Thus, though ambiguity is constituted by an ontological intertwining, harmony and care are not its necessary consequence. Willing the freedom of the other and acting to facilitate it constitutes an ethical decision, not an ontological necessity. Violence is also a possible response to the ontological *Mitsein*, and what makes violence so terribly destructive is this original, indissoluble "me-other" link: others give me life and meaning, but they can also oppress, objectify, or destroy me at any moment.[11] Neoliberal conceptions of a subject that is sovereign, independent, and free from others thus seem, from the perspective of Beauvoir's philosophy, like mere fantasies, probably constructed as protection from the inherent ambiguity (and fragility) of our existence. If we do not want to submit to bad faith, we must recognize that we are more knotted together with others than separate from them. Langer writes, regarding Beauvoir's and Merleau-Ponty's shared ontology: "Unlike pure consciousnesses, we 'blend' with, and compose, a common situation—an intersubjectivity. Further, we feel the need for others' recognition" (Langer 2003, 101).

From Beauvoir's Ambiguity to Butler's Vulnerability

Murphy (2011; 2012) rightly considers Beauvoir's ambiguity the most obvious predecessor of Butler's vulnerability. According to Murphy, it was Beauvoir who first moved "from a descriptive ontology of vulnerability to a normative ethics" (Murphy 2012, 107). It was Beauvoir who recognized that because we are ontologically ambiguous, we are ontologically vulnerable, and therefore always potentially open to violence as well as to solidarity and care (though never necessarily to any of them). Thus, Murphy considers recent feminist conceptualizations of vulnerability—such as Butler's—as originating from Beauvoir's ontology of ambiguity.[12] Butler's vulnerability, like Beauvoir's ambiguity, describes an ontological reality of inherent connection and interdependence that opens a pathway to myriad normative reactions, including rampant violence, indifference, and oppression. Butler discusses embodied vulnerability as a phenomenological condition revealing our individual selves as not individual at all but constituted by support and relationships that, when denied or broken, expose a "specific vulnerability":

> We cannot talk about a body without knowing what supports that body and what its relation to that support—or lack of support—might be. In this way, *the body is less an entity than a relation*, and it cannot be fully dissociated from the infrastructural and environmental conditions of its living. Thus, the dependency of human and other creatures on infrastructural support exposes a *specific vulnerability* that we have when we are unsupported, when those infrastructural conditions characterizing our social, political, and economic lives start to decompose, or when we find ourselves radically unsupported under conditions of precarity or under explicit conditions of threat.
>
> (Butler 2016, 19; emphasis added)

Following Beauvoir's and Butler's ideas, Murphy argues for a positive feminist recognition of vulnerability and interdependence as a way to counter the negative evaluation of these concepts under patriarchy and the correspondingly overly positive patriarchal assessments of autonomy and independence, which fail to recognize our true relational being-in-the-world:

> *there is a sense in which the body we defend as our own can never be only that.* As embodied, we are necessarily exposed to others; we struggle for recognition, and suffer for the lack thereof. Hence while feminist theorists acknowledge the importance of claims to bodily integrity, they also suggest there must be another normative

> aspiration that rests alongside these claims of autonomy and self-determination. *Claims to autonomy and integrity must be coincident with the acknowledgment we are radically dependent on others for the formation and persistence of our social selves.*
>
> (Murphy 2009, 58; emphasis added)

Violence is not overcome by denying or suppressing vulnerability and ambiguity or by emphasizing freedom and sovereignty. Violence is always a possibility—sometimes even necessary, per Beauvoir. But it is precisely by recognizing our vulnerable and ambiguous ontological condition—our inherent embodiment, attachment, and need of others—that we can allow an ethics of care and solidarity to flourish.

Thus, for a more accurate, more productive critique of obstetric violence, we must think about our phenomenological condition more in terms of connections and support than through concepts like bodily integrity or self-determination; consequently, we must recognize obstetric violence primarily as violence that prevents connection and care. This might also entail a shift in the form of our activism and policies against obstetric violence, emphasizing a feminist struggle for support and affective care rather than independence and freedom (Herring 2013; Herring 2019; Herring 2020).

Conclusions: Rethinking Obstetric Violence through Ambiguity and Vulnerability

Let us not essentialize laboring bodies. They are not always powerful, loud, or expansive. Recalling her own labors, Rich writes: "A part of me, even then, could not tolerate passivity, but I identified that part with the 'unwomanly' and in becoming a mother I was trying to affirm myself as a 'womanly woman.' If passivity was required, I would conform myself to the expectation" (Rich 1986, 129).

Martin (2003) argues that white, middle-class, heterosexual women giving birth in capitalist Western societies are characterized by hesitation and a general desire to be polite. Using Young's (1980) analysis, however, Martin shows that this attitude may well originate in women's internalization of certain (repressive, censoring) feminine comportment norms. We could see Young's ideas as preceding Martin's argument: the hesitation of these women in labor could be seen as a (mostly unconscious) way to head off the violence that might otherwise be used to domesticate them. Laboring bodies are at least potentially perceived as antithetical to the myth of femininity, undermining the feminine mode of bodily comportment under patriarchy, and thus threatening hegemonic power. Violence, then, seems necessary in order to domesticate these bodies, make them "feminine" again. Women might well want to avoid this violence by approaching childbirth through an already hesitant, docile, silent body. Preemptively becoming feminine might save us from being put in our place by others.

This is of course not a real solution. Women must be able to labor authentically as part of living authentically; we should be able to experience ourselves integrally, as fully embodied subjectivities free from objectifying violence or coercive practices, in labor and beyond. One of the things that most haunts me from my last labor is that even in my pain and confusion, I understood that I was living a unique moment of potential loud, forceful, embodied authenticity, yet this moment was taken from me in a strikingly violent, humiliating way, transformed into an oppressive "I cannot." Identifying violence in labor as part of not just the medical objectification of patients but the general violence used to domesticate and silence women and their bodies under patriarchy will open new spaces for discussion, leading to real changes in obstetric practices and how women can experience labor.

Childbirth is, also, a social event, usually experienced with others, who constitute a meaningful part of the experience. Beauvoir recognized the importance of company in childbirth, even calling this need vital, proof of our ambiguous condition as both part of nature and socially and culturally constructed. Discussing childbirth in *The Second Sex*, she argues:

> What is significant is that normally woman—like some domesticated female animals—*needs help to accomplish the function to which nature destines her*; there are peasants in rough conditions and shamed young unmarried mothers who give birth alone: but their solitude often brings about the death of the child or for the mother incurable illnesses. At the very moment woman completes the realization of her feminine destiny, she is still dependent: which also proves that in the human species nature can never be separated from artifice.
>
> (Beauvoir 2011, 547–548; emphasis added)[13]

LaChance Adams and Burcher (2014) further emphasize the shared and social aspect of childbirth when analyzing the strange phenomenon of "communal pushing" in childbirth and explaining how the ambiguous "intersubjective body" (Merleau-Ponty 1995 [1945])—which is "both distinct and prereflectively united to others" (Adams and Burcher 2014, 73)—might help to describe it. Significant others present at childbirth push with the laboring woman, adding themselves to her pushing, supporting her in her efforts without even reflecting on this. The woman is never lost in the others, however; she is always singular, a subject—*the* laboring subject—and she is always "the hardest pusher" (Adams and Burcher 2014, 76):

> the communal push represents support without a complete loss of body identity. That is, the body understands it is creating a shared space in which the pushing woman feels that others are focusing with her on the task that is still ultimately hers alone … But the sharing that occurs includes a "forgetting" of a place—a partial *loss* of individuality. Indeed, when people are made aware of the fact that they are pushing with the woman in labor, they generally stop pushing, at least for a time. We find that communal pushing … exemplifies the complexity of human intersubjectivity, the way in which interweaving is both ubiquitous and unique, each individual responding differently to the bodily need of another … This sharing does include the potential for bodies to care for one another in ways that actually *move* us at the prereflective level.
>
> (Adams and Burcher 2014, 76, 78; emphasis in the original)

This intersubjectivity—childbirth's shared and communal character, which Beauvoir noticed and that communal pushing strikingly exemplifies—is truncated, even destroyed, by obstetric violence. It is precisely this ambiguous character of childbirth that can turn labor into a powerful experience of caring and solidarity and, at the same time, puts laboring women in serious danger of undergoing violence. Birthing women are (both *inherently* and *situationally*) especially vulnerable, even if they are also, frequently, particularly strong and loud.

The laboring body is notably susceptible to violence mainly because it is not alone: because we (usually) birth with others. But coping with obstetric violence—making birth humane, respected, even empowering—cannot involve denying the intersubjectivity of birth by exclusively or predominantly emphasizing the birthing woman's agency, independence, and freedom. It is instead by revealing and fostering childbirth's interpersonal, shared, communal character that we might discover solutions to the urgent problem of obstetric violence.

Notes

1 This is how we gain authentic subjectivity, according to Beauvoir, who writes that "every existent is simultaneously immanence and transcendence" (Beauvoir 2011, 316). In order to recognize this ambiguity as pertaining to all subjects, she argues, we must first recognize ourselves as ambiguous: not only free, transcendent subjectivities projected into the future but also embedded in otherness. The task is to identify ourselves as freedom while simultaneously recognizing the otherness within us, fleshing out and embodying our own immanence (Beauvoir 1948, 102–103). I provided a Beauvoirian analysis of birth as transcendent and immanent in Cohen Shabot (2017b). In the following, I deal with Beauvoir's idea of ambiguity in more detail.

2 "Autonomy" is not only or always constructed as emphasizing freedom from others, free will, and individual agency, but this is the "autonomy" that has prevailed in discussions of obstetric violence. The following accounts, on which I base my new understanding of the ills of obstetric violence, do not deny the idea of autonomy but provide resources for thinking about it differently, mainly as achieved through and together with others—as "relational." I deal more thoroughly with the idea of "relational autonomy" below.

3 Wagner for instance, considers medicalized birth *necessarily* dehumanizing because "in medicalized birth the doctor is always in control while the key element in humanized birth is the woman in control of her own birthing and whatever happens to her" (Wagner 2001, S26), while Smeenk and ten Have see the problem in medicalized pregnancy and childbirth mainly as related to depriving birthing subjects of autonomy in the sense of voiding their independence and freedom of choice:

> "Discussing medicalization of pregnancy and childbirth, moral problems concerning the autonomy of the pregnant women arise. *The core element in defining autonomy is independence: freedom to choose …* By expanding professional power over gestation and birth, the number of options seems to have increased. Therefore, autonomy apparently is enhanced. However, this development is a mixed blessing: the options within the wider area of non-medical as well as medical approaches are increasingly replaced by more options within only the much smaller area of medical science. Thus, the quantity of options is increased but

> the quality reduced. We can choose among more of the same options within the domain of medical approaches. Can we really maintain that autonomy is enhanced if medical options are expanded while at the same time the idea of pregnancy and birth as physiological processes is discarded as irrelevant?" (Smeenk and ten Have 2003, 162; emphasis added)

4 Chadwick (2017) argues similarly for the necessity of reconceptualizing obstetric violence, proposing a Foucauldian framework. Chadwick emphasizes the need to see obstetric violence as relational, disciplinary, and productive of a certain ambiguous agency for women. She advocates recognizing obstetric violence as structural, not behavioral: layered, immersed in complex, subtle, frequently still-unacknowledged relations of power. My arguments respond to her proposal that more nuanced accounts of the phenomenon be pursued.

5 Some women decide to give birth unattended by doctors or midwives (either with their partners or completely alone). These are not the births that I mean by "solitary births." A woman who chooses to birth unassisted and expects no assistance or care from staff is not disappointed at the lack of assistance. Such a decision to birth unattended (Miller 2009; Miller 2012; Shanley 2012), however, is still marginal and uncommon. Miller notices the influence of neoliberal ideals of "individualism" and "freedom" on some of the women choosing unassisted births, who consider the most empowering option to be a labor completely on their terms, without help from others (Miller 2009, 53).

6 Since I am examining the *phenomenology* of obstetric violence—more women's perceptions and experiences than formal definitions—I use research on traumatic labor (not just strictly obstetric violence) to make my point about how we might better conceive of obstetric violence. Not all violent childbirths result in trauma for the laboring woman; the research shows that such trauma is mostly associated with how labor develops and specific interactions with the medical staff, rather than with the results of the birth, horrific as these can be (Simpson and Catling 2015). In their study of traumatic births, Elmir et al. conclude:

> "Our findings indicate that women are often traumatized as a result of the actions or inactions of midwives, nurses and doctors. The care received was sometimes experienced as dehumanizing, disrespectful and uncaring … Women who report high levels of dissatisfaction with labour and birth care commonly describe midwives and other professionals as unhelpful, insensitive, abrupt and rude" (Elmir et al. 2010, 2150)

This is why I assume that most traumatic births are in some way violent.

7 On the necessary connection between authenticity and ethics in Beauvoir see, for instance, Cohen Shabot and Menschenfreund (2008).

8 Beauvoir's idea of ambiguity has been thoroughly analyzed; see Bergoffen (1997), Gothlin (2006), Heinämaa (2003), Keltner (2006), Kruks (2012), Langer (2003), and Murphy (2012).

9 On Merleau-Ponty's ontology as an influence on Beauvoir see Heinämaa (2003), Langer (2003), and McWeeny (2017). Langer in particular deals with the similarities between Merleau-Ponty's and Beauvoir's ideas of ambiguity. On Merleau-Ponty's and Beauvoir's shared ontology of embodied intersubjectivity as necessarily calling for an ethical standpoint, McWeeny writes: "An ontology that acknowledges that a body is always in contact with a world and with others also announces our capacity to affect one another and to be responsible for each other" (McWeeny 2017, 215).

10 The readings of Bauer (2006) and Gothlin (2003) interpret the *Mitsein* in Beauvoir as exclusively describing an ontological reality, never calling for a specific ethics. Bergoffen (1997), however, does recognize the Beauvoirian *Mitsein* as posing ethical demands.

11 Sometimes, according to Beauvoir, violence is actually necessary. This is part of Beauvoir's ambiguity: violence is not always an evil. In the face of a freedom that is only used to take another's freedom, violence is justified: "We have to respect freedom only when it is intended for freedom, not when it strays, flees itself, and resigns itself. A freedom which is interested only in denying freedom must be denied" (Beauvoir 1948, 90–91). See also Kruks (2012) and Murphy (2011; 2012), especially the last chapter of Kruks on revenge in Beauvoir's thought.

12 Some feminist discussions of vulnerability expose the danger of marking vulnerability as positive with regard to women: emphasizing women's vulnerability can risk fostering inequality by justifying paternalistic, controlling, and oppressive practices towards women when they appear in extraordinary need of protection (Herring 2020; Mackenzie et al. 2014, 6). However, the feminist elaborations of vulnerability that I use here—considering vulnerability an ontological given for all subjects—not only avoid the risk of recognizing women as especially vulnerable and thus particularly needing protection, but can in fact serve as an antidote to traditional, patriarchal conceptions of vulnerability. Neither Beauvoir nor Butler considers women *inherently* more vulnerable than men. Women might be more vulnerable due to specific oppressive circumstances (they might suffer from *situational* vulnerability) that should be opposed and contested—but never by denying ontological vulnerability. (On inherent versus situational vulnerability see Mackenzie et al. 2014, 7.) Vulnerability being an ontological condition shared by all, it is not paternalistic protection we need but rather a mutual recognition of our inherent interdependence, along with nonhierarchical ways to cope with it—as I will show, relying on Murphy.

For a compelling account of vulnerability in feminist theory and the debates surrounding its advantages and disadvantages for feminist purposes, see Mackenzie et al. (2014); Rogers (2014); and Rogers et al. (2012).

13 Beauvoir even recognizes here that childbirth might, in certain cases, be experienced as a creative, powerful act—even sensually pleasurable—offering a remarkable report of one such case. This report includes a description of the fairly sexual experience that the laboring woman undergoes, through embodied contact with her midwife: "I am so strongly sexed that even childbirth means to me a sexual act … I had a very pretty 'madame' for a nurse. She bathed me and gave me my vaginal douches. This was enough for me—it kept me in such a high state of sexual agitation that I trembled" (Beauvoir 2011, 549). Again, the social and intersubjective aspect of birth is emphasized here. For more on the sexual character of labor, see Cohen Shabot (2017a).

2 The Epistemological Perspective

Is This Violence? Gaslighting and Testimonial Injustice

In this chapter, I first examine the phenomenon of obstetric violence through the concept of "gaslighting." I argue that a central part of obstetric violence involves laboring women being disbelieved, distrusted, and (unjustifiably) questioned about their violent laboring experiences and even, more pressingly, made to doubt their own experiences and feel deprived of epistemic authority altogether. This distrust shown to laboring women operates both during and after labor, when they attempt to tell others about their (violent) laboring experiences and obtain epistemic recognition from these others. I emphasize that this experience of deep distrust must be recognized not simply as a response to obstetric violence but as a core component of the phenomenon.

The second part of the chapter deals with another form of epistemic injustice and its relation to obstetric violence.[1] This discussion focuses on developing a link between testimonial injustice in labor and the marked irrationality that is (sometimes rightly, sometimes mistakenly) seen as a core characteristic not only of women, or of marginalized subjects, but very specifically of birthing subjects—an irrationality that is always at odds with the kind of knowledge that is privileged within medicalized childbirth.

I use Fricker's analysis to argue that a central part of obstetric violence involves laboring women being "*wrongfully undermined specifically in … [their] capacity as knower[s]*" (Fricker 2007, 20; emphasis in the original): distrusted because of a double prejudice: first, deriving simply from their condition as women (a prejudice that is exacerbated in birth because of its strong historical and conceptual link to the uterus as responsible for women's irrationality[2]), and

DOI: 10.4324/9781003593829-3

second, involving the kind of knowledge that many women in fact find useful in the birthing process.

"But You Cannot Know For Sure, Can You?"

I have experienced several miscarriages. During one of them, I started bleeding when I was six weeks and five days into pregnancy. I went to the hospital, and was seen by a young female gynecologist. She seemed truly empathetic and kind. One of the first things she did, after briefly conversing with me and my partner, was to examine me via ultrasound. She saw a tiny sac, with an approximately four-week-old embryo, a discovery she communicated to me optimistically. "You are four weeks pregnant," she said, "and you are bleeding, like so many women at this stage. Everything seems to be all right; do not worry too much." "But there is no heartbeat," I countered. "Of course there isn't," she replied, immutable: "at four weeks we still cannot see any heartbeat." Then I started impatiently explaining to her, for a second time now, that I was in fact not four but rather almost seven weeks pregnant, and that this was surely an embryo that had stopped developing at four weeks (similarly to what happened to me in several past pregnancies). It was then that a patronizing dialogue of distrust began:

> "But you do not really know *exactly* when you got pregnant, do you?"
> "The truth is that I know the precise date," I responded.
> "But you cannot know *for sure,*" she continued.
> "I do believe I can, though: I feel ovulation very clearly and I also used an ovulation predictor kit."
> "Well, this is what I see in the ultrasound," she said, attempting to use technology, the ultimate silencing weapon, to bring this hierarchical conversation to a happy end.
> "You just do not believe me; you do not believe me at all, right?" I tried desperately, one last time.

She wielded her final condescending weapon: "Well, we cannot base a diagnosis on your intuitions, can we?" And then I just shut up. I knew this was pointless. I could not convince her. In her view, I was still pregnant. To me, it was clear that I was miscarrying. I had experience, and I had knowledge, but this knowledge was being mercilessly silenced and turned, by the "epistemic authority," into "pure intuition": just another suspicious female hunch, not to be trusted. Thus, as an adult woman in my forties, a responsible professional, a professor of philosophy, I was sent home and told not to worry, since in eight more months I would probably become a mother for the third time.

I went home, and I miscarried. Everything was all right, and I needed no further intervention, but that meeting with the kind doctor required reflection, especially because after I went home that night, before I miscarried, I had noted something else awakening in me alongside my anger and desperation at being disbelieved: namely self-distrust. I felt uneasy, no longer entirely sure whether I might not really be four weeks pregnant after all, instead of seven; not sure whether I knew anything at all for certain. In the end, I thought, it would be nice if she was right, and maybe she was, and, after all, how could I *really* know?[3]

Reflecting on this experience in retrospect, I could not help but notice the similarities it had with some of the forms of obstetric violence I had undergone in my second childbirth—which I documented and analyzed as examples of the broad experience of obstetric violence in my first paper on the subject. I suddenly understood that this experience of profound distrust and disbelief was a recurrent, aching theme in stories denouncing obstetric violence: women being infantilized and having our reports of pain or power—of knowing what our bodies were either suffering or enduring with strength during childbirth—be dismissed by medical authorities (whether doctors or nurses) in the labor room[4] and also, even more stressfully, by well-meaning allies listening to our labor experiences after the fact. But there was something else: this experience too often developed into one of self-distrust; it was eventually tainted by a disempowering feeling of deep self-doubt and, in consequence, of loss of autonomy.[5] In other words, in addition to being condescendingly questioned regarding our most intimate embodied experiences, we were ultimately being convinced that "they knew better"; we were truly made to feel and believe that we had been exaggerating: It even seemed somewhat reasonable to assume—precisely because of the pain of childbirth, because of our vulnerable state during it, because we were probably a little "hysterical"—that we had been magnifying "what everybody goes through" and making a fuss over a "normal" experience.[6] This is of course the ultimate silencing tool. It is one thing to know that our experiences are not trusted, but to be convinced to mistrust ourselves—to believe that we are indeed wrong, exaggerating, crazy, or ultimately not even capable of judging—is the most effective form of oppression. Such a deep internalization of self-distrust and of the belief that we are not worthy epistemic agents is the ultimate tool through which hegemonic powers can continue unquestioned and untouched.

I have come to understand that I, along with many other women, have been continuously gaslighted as a part of our experience of obstetric violence and our ensuing encounters with those to whom we tell our stories. In the following, I will use the concept of gaslighting as a way to account for this particular experience of self-distrust as a part of the scenarios of obstetric violence.

On Gaslighting

The 1944 film *Gaslight* tells the story of a man, Gregory, who attempts to drive his wife, Paula, crazy in order to obtain the jewels she inherited. As Gregory manipulates Paula, he gradually succeeds in making her doubt her own perceptions and distrust her own knowledge and judgment. Lately, "gaslighting" has been analyzed as a specific form of epistemic injustice, in which a (usually) more powerful person or group intentionally or unintentionally[7] causes a weaker one to distrust her/their own perceptions, thus further diminishing or oppressing the person or group that was weaker to begin with (Abramson 2014; Flores Ruíz 2014; McKinnon 2017).

Thus, in gaslighting, the victim is radically questioned: not only questioned for a particular belief but made to altogether doubt her own epistemic competence. Gaslighting usually involves others persistently distrusting her epistemic skills, and it is more effective when the gaslighters are indeed many, rather than one.

On Obstetric Violence as Gaslighting

The idea that certain instances of obstetric violence might be accurately explored through the concept of gaslighting definitively hit me when I read Abramson's phenomenological description of the feeling of being gaslighted:

> Think about one of your worst experiences, an experience which either itself, or in its effects, went on months. Now imagine that while you were going through that, all or most of the voices around

> you either flatly denied that anything worth being upset about was going on, or radically minimized it, or reconceptualized the experience so that it was not so uncomfortable (for them) to live with. You protested. The protestations were greeted with "that's crazy," "it's not a big deal," "you're overreacting." Somehow you endured. But the very fact of your survival then became woven in to the rewriting of history, to confirm the minimizing and denials and later repression. (E.g. "Well, you survived, didn't you?", "It all worked out in the end" or "That was just a minor blip.") So, at no point during it did someone (or perhaps someone, but not enough, or perhaps just not the people most dear to you) look at you and confirm the reality of horror with which you were dealing. To the contrary, they said you're crazy for being upset, oversensitive, and any difficulty you might have is "all in you." That's what gaslighting is like.
>
> (Abramson 2014, 5–6)

Gaslighting has been defined as being at least frequently sexist, although not inherently so (Abramson 2014, 3). It is particularly done to women, as a weaker group whose epistemic capacities have always been questioned anyway. Disbelief, to the point of silencing the victim by convincing her that she probably is crazy and what happened was not *that* terrible, is a constant in sexual violence. Rape victims are persistently disbelieved; their silences, for months and even years after the violent encounter, are due partly to shame, along with the certainty that their testimony will be questioned.[8] But the silence is often also due to the fact that when they did tell, they were gaslighted, and in consequence they feel that they no longer know whether what happened was really violent or really important.

In order to understand gaslighting as part of obstetric violence, it is important to understand obstetric violence, again, as a kind of gender violence. In the labor room, women are gaslighted by the staff, which frequently casts doubt on their pain, their capacity for laboring, and/or their knowledge of their own bodily processes. In her description of power relations in American maternity wards, Jordan (1997) offers a concrete example of this typical underestimation of women's knowledge in labor. Jordan describes a particular case in which the woman is infantilized and "not allowed" to push until the doctor comes into the room and confirms that she is ready:

> She knows she has to push and says so clearly. She also expresses it in the visible, almost superhuman effort she marshals to suppress the urge to push. But every time she tries to get her desire—her expressed knowledge about the state of her body—acknowledged and made the basis for proceeding with the birth, her version of reality is overridden, is ignored, is denied, or, most frequently, is sidetracked, deflected, and replaced with some other definition of reality. Something else is offered up as being more relevant, as might happen to an obstinate child whose parent opts for distraction rather than confrontation.
>
> (Jordan 1997, 67)

Once the labor is done, victims of obstetric violence often encounter harsh interlocutors who use "At least you have a healthy baby" as the ultimate response, to erase and silence any further complaints about the violent labor or the physical and emotional trauma it left behind. Countless women undergo gaslighting at the hands of their own natural allies: their most loved ones, their partners, women friends who have recently given birth, their mothers, their health care providers. This gaslighting is most often unconsciously perpetrated, due at least partially to the normalization of violent practices in childbirth and the internalization of the idea that birthing women are only vessels for their babies and should be willing to sacrifice themselves for them, as "good" mothers do: that they should be thankful just to have survived childbirth along with their babies.

Thus, because suffering is perceived as integral to childbirth, and childbirth is considered a routine, even compulsory, process for women, the painful and violent experiences of laboring women go unrecognized by both the women's immediate community and the medical staff. New mothers who share traumatic, or even simply difficult, birth stories are silenced with comments like "everybody goes through that," "you should be grateful," or the abovementioned "all that matters is that the baby is healthy." This is how gaslighting shames, disciplines, and silences birthing mothers. Humphries's blog (2001) recounts the responses to her attempts to tell people about the trauma she experienced after undergoing a violent emergency Caesarean section:

> Wasn't I grateful? So many people said it to me, I started to wonder. People I trusted, people I respected, people I loved. Maybe I wasn't

> grateful for my babies? Maybe I didn't love my babies as much as I should or as much as other mothers did? … I didn't *feel* a lot about them. I was depressed.[9]
>
> (Humphries 2001; emphasis in the original)

The gaslighting of birthing women is possible because it takes place within a general context in which women are considered to be already flawed epistemic agents or not epistemic agents at all. Jordan (1997), in a study that has become a classic and that remains relevant and essentially unchallenged still today, describes power relations in the American hospital labor room as clearly privileging the knowledge of doctors over that of nurses, and the knowledge of nurses over that of the laboring woman, thus putting her at the bottom of the epistemic hierarchy:

> [In] American hospital births … medical knowledge supersedes and delegitimizes other potentially relevant sources of knowledge such as the woman's prior experience and the knowledge she has of the state of her body. Nonmedical knowledge is devalued by all participants, usually including the woman herself, who comes to believe that the course charted on the basis of professional medical knowledge is the best for her … In the labor room, authoritative knowledge is privileged, the prerogative of the physician, without whose official certification of the woman's state the birth cannot proceed.
>
> (Jordan 1997, 61, 64)

The dismissal of women's knowledge and understanding of women as flawed epistemic agents extends beyond the realm of medicine or medicalized childbirth. Feminist epistemological theories show that underestimating women's knowledge has been a pervasive motif within patriarchy and is not merely circumstantial. Women's knowledge has generally been considered unreliable and inferior, mainly because its origins are supposedly more emotional and less rational (Jaggar 1989; Lloyd 1984).

How the quality of knowledge is measured is, thus, itself a product of power relations: certain kinds of knowledge have been privileged not because of any true correspondence with reality but rather out of sexist, racist, and classist prejudices.[10]

Thus, we are gaslighted in the ob-gyn office, in the labor room, and when recounting our violent childbirth experiences, as part of a general devaluation of women's epistemological capacities and of the hegemonic patriarchal culture, which is sexist and misogynistic to the core. But if obstetric violence is the dehumanization and objectification of women within obstetric practices, if it means infantilizing us and depriving us of agency and autonomy over our birthing bodies, then this form of gaslighting must be recognized as obstetric violence too.

My own story here has a happy ending: I contacted the young doctor after I miscarried, writing her in detail about what finally happened and explaining to her why her distrust had been painful to me and how it made me doubt my own knowledge. I told her that I believed this to be a form of obstetric violence, and I sent her my paper on the subject. She read, and reflected, and her views changed. She has since become one of the researchers and activists against obstetric violence within the medical system, and we are currently working together on common projects. But this only happened because I was a relatively privileged victim of gaslighting; because gaslighting did not, in fact, really work in my case. It also happened because the truly privileged epistemic status-holder in this event was ready to listen and to think critically about her own position of power.

Women as Flawed Epistemic Agents

From the broader perspective of the epistemologies of injustice, Fricker (2007) reinforces the feminist theories of epistemology that describe the pervasive underestimation of women's knowledge. Fricker's theory of testimonial injustice is most useful in addressing, specifically, the pervasive disbelief and distrust of birthing women's voices. Fricker explains testimonial injustice as an "agential operation of social power" (Fricker 2007, 12), characterized by the devaluation of the knowledge of a certain subject (suffering from a credibility deficit) by a listener, with no other justification than the listener's underlying prejudice.

"Systematic testimonial injustice," specifically, is not an incidental prejudice but a "negative identity prejudice," in which it is the whole identity of the subject that lacks credibility, not simply one specific situation where this subject is considered incompetent. Women, for instance, are disenfranchised as a group and suffer from systematic testimonial injustice, their knowledge generally considered problematic or less authoritative, rendering them vulnerable to many other, additional injustices.

This argument is reminiscent of previous feminist epistemological arguments about the pervasive devaluation of women's epistemic capacities. Yet, alongside this pervasive "systematic testimonial injustice," Fricker also finds it important to deal with a less severe form of testimonial injustice—the incidental. Here the whole subject is not doubted or unrecognized as epistemically authoritative, but the type of knowledge she brings to a specific situation is contested:

> There are all sorts of prejudices that can cause credibility deficit, yet where the resultant testimonial injustice is highly localized and therefore lacking any … structural social significance … Imagine, for instance … a panel of referees on a science journal who have **a dogmatic prejudice against a certain research method**. It might reasonably be complained by a would-be contributor that authors who present hypotheses on the basis of the disfavoured method receive a prejudicially reduced level of credibility from the panel. Thus the prejudice is such as to generate a genuine testimonial injustice (writing being one medium of testimony). Although such a testimonial injustice may be grievous for the careers of the would-be contributors, and perhaps even for the progress of science, none the less its impact on the subject's life is, let us assume, highly localized. That is to say, the prejudice in question (against a certain scientific method) does not render the subject vulnerable to any other kinds of injustice (legal, economic, political). Let us say that the testimonial injustice produced here is *incidental*.
>
> (Fricker 2007, 27; italic emphasis in the original, bold emphasis added)

While the subject experiencing testimonial injustice suffers a credibility deficit, there is a parallel subject who profits unjustifiably from credibility excess: who is believed, due to prejudice, to know more than he does. Interestingly, Fricker gives the example of a general medical practitioner, believed by his patients to have more epistemic power than he actually does.

I argue that while laboring women clearly suffer from systematic testimonial injustice, due to the pervasive prejudice against women as epistemic subjects, the incidental form of testimonial injustice deriving from medicalized childbirth's prejudice against the specific kind of knowledge that women bring to labor is also important. To paraphrase Fricker: many birthing women appear to the medical staff to be going about their labor "incorrectly." Labor, consequently, becomes an especially damaging arena, where women suffer from these two forms of testimonial injustice added to each other, while medical practitioners enjoy a credibility excess.

Systematic Testimonial Injustice in the Labor Room

Birthing women of all kinds, including privileged women, are systematically disbelieved as part of the structural mechanisms that allow obstetric violence. Thus, testimonial injustice in childbirth is part of the systematic testimonial injustice inflicted on women within patriarchy (see Fricker 2007). I argue that testimonial injustice in childbirth is part of a systematic injustice, deeply linked to the pervasive distrust of women's knowledge and epistemic capacities generally and within medical settings in particular.[11] Moreover, labor and the labor room constitute a very special terrain, since the implicit bias that women are less rational than men or lack certain epistemic capacities is historically grounded in ideas about the uterus and women's reproductive systems as key to women's irrationality.[12] This bias is reinforced by the overly embodied "scene" of labor: women's bodies, specifically their reproductive and sexual embodied features, are, indeed, "excessively" present in labor (Cohen Shabot 2016; Cohen Shabot 2017a) and are taken to obscure women's rational capacities even more than in "normal" situations. Laboring women may be considered even more clearly (more so than within disease, and definitely more so than in situations involving neither disease nor labor) driven by their bodies, their sexuality, their "irrational" uteruses, and thus even more irrational than common patriarchal constructions already consider them: in other words, if women in medicalized settings are more prone than men to encounter disbelief and distrust, and if this distrust results from their being perceived as less rational and more emotional, then women's "excessively-driven-by-their-uteruses" situation during labor only accentuates this tendency. Current testimonies by women reveal that women's voices in childbirth remain untrusted and contested to this day.[13]

Testimonial injustice during childbirth, thus, results from the systematic consideration of women as flawed epistemic agents. But behind this notorious dismissal of women's voices, ideas, and desires in labor lie important unexamined assumptions about what constitutes "knowledge" in labor and who is recognized as possessing that knowledge. This is why testimonial injustice in labor also constitutes a case of incidental testimonial injustice (Fricker 2007), as I discuss next.

Incidental Testimonial Injustice: What Do We Talk About When We Talk About Knowledge in Labor?

Edwards (2005), writing about women's birthing autonomy during planned home births, analyzes the particular dismissal of women's knowledge in pregnancy and labor as directly connected to the common patriarchal dismissal of emotions and embodied sensations as proper knowledge:

> Those who believe that pure male reason, free of all emotion and any other so-called distractions, is the only sound basis for producing knowledge, will also believe that women's knowledge is unreliable and lacking. This kind of thinking dismisses women's knowledge about themselves and their experiences, and undermines the knowledge they have. For example, several of the women I talked to *knew* when they had conceived, but were disbelieved… . Privileging rationality over emotion and the mind over the body vastly reduces what counts as knowledge, because it prevents women's experiences, for example, from being part of that knowledge.
>
> (Edwards 2005, 51–52; emphasis added)[14]

Jordan (1997) describes power relations in American hospital labor rooms where laboring women are at the bottom of the epistemic hierarchy, as we have seen, and technology is clearly considered the most reliable source of knowledge (always more reliable than a woman's voice or embodied experience, and usually inaccessible to her). "Woman's knowledge counts for nothing," Jordan bluntly explains.

Thus, the medicalized model of childbirth turns birthing women into passive objects. Their knowledge, Jordan reminds us, is nothing but a burden to the staff: untranslatable into charts or medical information, this knowledge—including previous experience, sensations, bodily transformations, and reactions—is only distracting, useless noise.[15]

The medical practitioners attending hospital births therefore enjoy an unjust excess of credibility (Fricker 2007), while birthing women suffer not only testimonial injustice derived from general systematic prejudices against their epistemic capacities, but also incidental testimonial injustice, the devaluation of the specific type of knowledge many of them bring into labor because it is achieved through a "flawed" method. Not only is this knowledge devalued, but women frequently encounter violence when they try to use it: they are punished, humiliated, even persecuted for daring to labor outside of the system's norms (or outside the system completely, as with unassisted births).[16] Reed argues that women are judged for laboring loudly or "out of control." In this way, paradoxically, they are frequently prevented from laboring efficiently:

> In fact it seems that being quiet and "controlled" is considered to be the best way to birth. How many times have you heard a woman's labour described in a positive way because she was "so in control and quietly breathed her baby out"? In contrast, the loud woman is encouraged to breathe (ie. stop screaming/shouting) and focus … These women are often described as "not coping"—when in fact they are coping just fine … but loudly. It is those around them who are not coping. Michel Odent suggests that the intense fear and sense of "losing it" often experienced near the end of labour [i.e. if labor is not medically controlled] facilitates the fetal ejection reflex. Not many women experience this because midwives (or others) intervene to calm the woman and help her gain control of herself.
>
> (Reed 2011)

Questions of authority and trust in childbirth are, thus, epistemic questions. They concern how we construct and refer to knowledge. They are deeply connected to what we think knowledge is. When we take medical authority as given, and medical knowledge as indisputable—the only right knowledge for managing childbirth—a woman's knowledge of her birthing body (and of birth traditions, others' birth experiences, her intuition, etc.) is automatically dismissed. But objectively speaking, knowledge around birth is not solely, or even mainly, the possession of doctors or medical staff: women have knowledge—at least some—of their bodies, their birthing processes; and doctors frequently lack knowledge of nonmedicalized physiological birth.

Doctors, trained to spot pathology, are less acquainted with birth as a normal physiological process, and this ignorance produces the most significant kinds of damage done by the medicalization of childbirth. Thus the injustice in the labor room is also incidental, because women giving birth with little or no intervention, who frequently act in ways recalling wild, animal-like behavior, including bodily noises, grunts, and secretions, expressing an open, indomitable embodied self, are punished for this behavior, which is incompatible with medicalized paradigms of knowledge and expectations of measurable, controllable processes.

Dahan (2019; 2020; 2021a) makes a strong case for the hypothesis that women's brains during unmedicated, undisturbed labor act similarly to how they do in situations where rationality has been proven to be put aside, at least momentarily, while other states of consciousness prevail. Does this mean that during childbirth, women are less suited to making reliable decisions? Dahan's extremely original studies propose that the laboring brain appears to be both less rational *and* in control, and definitely a reliable source of knowledge during the birthing process. From her examinations of a significant amount of qualitative data on women's childbirth experiences and behavior, Dahan concludes that the states of consciousness developed during undisturbed, unmedicalized, physiological childbirth are very similar to the "transient-hypofrontality" produced by certain drugs, deep meditation, or hypnosis. In such a state, the more rational parts of our brains are temporarily put aside and neocortical activity is reduced, allowing less rational, less inhibited parts to predominate. This state is far from detrimental to a woman in labor. On the contrary: Dahan sees this state of consciousness as crucially enabling and supporting normal birth.

Finally, Dahan shows, it is when a woman feels compelled by others and is afraid and overwhelmed that she feels less in control and labor is more stressful; when a woman feels supported and contained, she experiences more control, even within her submission to pain and her irrationality.[17] But I must emphasize that this description does not apply to all women: those who opt for a highly medicalized birth from the start might, for instance, never experience the "irrational brain" during labor. And because not all women experience that, it is clearly the sexist prejudice about women's general irrationality that informs testimonial injustice in childbirth, regardless of the given laboring woman's actual state of consciousness. Therefore, this is mainly a case of systematic, rather than incidental, testimonial injustice.

Testimonial Injustice and the Question of "Correct" Knowledge in Childbirth

Testimonial injustice is a moral evil; in childbirth, it has the power to make a woman's labor a violent, traumatic experience. As we have seen, two main kinds of prejudice underlie the rampant testimonial injustice that laboring women suffer. The first is *systematic*, deriving from the fact that they are women, suffering a priori from lack of credibility and of epistemic authority, as part of their disenfranchisement under patriarchy and their supposed irrationality (as we learn from Fricker 2007, and others). In addition, birthing women are regarded as emphatically irrational because overtly embodied, mostly controlled by their reproductive functions (even more than in the general stereotype about women), thus unsuiting them for rational decisions. The second kind is *incidental*, involving the specific state of consciousness prevalent during physiological birth: an embodied knowledge, less rationally driven, less inhibited, more emotional, that challenges medical paradigms and biases but allows many women to birth securely and effectively.

The understanding of laboring women as irrational and "out of control"—reminiscent of nonhuman mammals or beasts—brings with it a concern about women's status as full subjects, as agents: this is one danger in relegating women to the realm of the natural and negating their right to freely and consciously decide about their own embodied selves (Martin 1987). But this is only relevant if rationally achieved knowledge is the only kind of knowledge that is recognized and irrationality is conflated with "animality": with weakness, lack of control, and inability to make correct decisions. Meanwhile, (feminist and other) phenomenological theories of embodied knowledge, of the body as a legitimate knowledge producer, along with recent hypotheses on the "birthing brain," demonstrate how inappropriate that would be. Birthing women have been shown to possess embodied knowledge that allows them to be in control, take optimal decisions, and birth efficiently.

While many women in medicalized labor settings suffer from the prejudice that women, because of their supposed irrationality, are per se defective epistemic subjects, the less "rational" mode of consciousness that these women are using in fact seems to allow them to birth more easily and successfully. Therefore, it may indeed be that the kind of knowledge that frequently guides birthing subjects (birthing physiologically, free from unnecessary interventions) is not primarily rationally driven. If so, then the injustice lies not in considering laboring women to be irrational but in failing to recognize certain irrational modes of consciousness and behavior as legitimate and useful in childbirth.

I want to stress that even if we found proof that laboring women were unable to make decisions based on reliable knowledge, that would not be a reason to dismiss their voices. Everyone deserves respect, autonomy, and humane care, whether or not their decisions are based on reliable knowledge. Women are always qualified to make decisions about their bodies; that should be their uncontested prerogative. But laboring women are disbelieved mostly because they are women, and because the kind of knowledge they frequently find productive in labor is not a kind that medical authorities recognize as legitimate or valuable—rather than because they are consistently mistaken in their practices or their judgment.

Notes

1 This discussion inserts itself into a recently developing broader feminist theorization of violence generally and gender violence particularly. Intention has frequently been considered a necessary part of violence properly defined (Landau 2010). More recent conceptualizations, however—mainly feminist ones, infused with Foucauldian interpretations and often also heavily relying on phenomenological accounts—discuss violence as pervasive within modern capitalist, patriarchal societies, where embodied subjects are disciplined through "invisible" violence, often with no clear intention on the perpetrator's part and not necessarily including physical harm (Butler 2004; Butler 2020; Mardorossian 2014; Murphy 2012, Taylor 2018). The invisibility of this violence makes it hard to recognize even for its victims. Current theorizations of violence address the important ontological, epistemological, and ethical philosophical problems this raises, making it clear that violence always demands to be discussed in the context of power relations and the epistemic obstacles to recognizing it. But the research is far from complete, and this chapter contributes to the particular discussion of gaslighting and testimonial injustice as epistemic violence, within the broader phenomenon of obstetric violence.

2 For more on labor as an event where women are seen as less rational, more animal, and less in control than the patriarchal narrative already considers them, because their uteruses and reproductive systems are central to the event, see Villarmea (2020); Villarmea and Kelly (2020). I will return to this argument and its consequences for epistemic authority in childbirth.

3 There are striking similarities between my case and the one described by McLeod (2002) in her chapter on miscarriages and self-distrust. She quotes a paper telling the story of Janet, who precisely and accurately

charted her first pregnancy and miscarried at seven and a half weeks of gestation:

> "Every morning the bleeding stopped and every afternoon it started and on the Wednesday we went back to our doctor. He felt, palpated, and prodded and questioned that I had ever been pregnant at all: 'You told me you were pregnant and I believed you.' *And I, knowing that I had been pregnant, started to doubt myself and my knowledge of my body.* I felt concerned for the doctor, that he felt he had made a mistake, and it was my fault. You are very willing to believe everything is your fault … I was afraid that the whole episode had just been hysteria, and he (the GP) was thinking 'neurotic woman.' … [Janet then explained that she had an ultrasound that confirmed her pregnancy.] … *I had known that I was pregnant, and I had doubted it, doubted me, doubted this little baby existence because some forms of knowledge are seen as more valid than others*" (Hey et al. 1996, cited in McLeod 2002, 38; emphasis added).

4 The internet is full of such reports these days. The Facebook page "Birth Monopoly," for instance, offers dozens of reports of women being mocked and patronized for bringing birth plans to their births. One such account reads:

> "My first birth I handed over my birth plan and the nurse literally LOL'd and said to the other nurse 'Look. First time mom with a birth plan *laughs*' I was openly disrespected. I should have walked right out of that hospital and checked in somewhere else. The nurse mocked me for going pain med free, didn't believe me when I told her I was about to vomit, didn't believe me when I told her my water had broken. She was awful. My OB was so respectful, though. I didn't get anything in my birth plan (ended with a c-section after my cervix swelled), but I knew that was likely. That nurse made my birth experience traumatic. Not the c-section, the nurse did" (Anonymous post on Pascucci, "Birth Monopoly," Facebook page, November 14, 2017).

5 On self-distrust as eventually leading to loss of autonomy, see McLeod (2002). McLeod considers self-trust in patients to be the result of an intersubjective, relational process in which the patient trusts her healthcare provider and in consequence trusts herself and is able to make autonomous decisions about her own health. Referring to one particular case, she writes:

> "Lee was not able to trust her health care providers to interpret the expression of her needs as legitimate, and as a result, she was not always able to trust herself to act in her own interests. Patients cannot trust themselves to be autonomous if they cannot trust physicians to give them room to express their autonomous desires, and also to inform them accurately about their health and health care options. Patient self-trust does not replace the need for trust between patients and practitioners" (McLeod 2002, 6).

6 For more on the phenomenon of distrusting women in medical settings, mainly with respect to the reproductive process, because of sexist assumptions that women are oversensitive, overly emotional, and epistemologically and morally incompetent in consequence, see for instance McLeod (2002, 8–9).

> Added to these sexist assumptions about women are assumptions about parenthood being a stressful and vulnerable condition, all of which assumptions are put onto women as they are going through the processes involved in becoming or trying to become mothers. Goering, for instance, writes about the experience of new parents in France when their babies are being taken care of in the newborn intensive care unit: "[They] are often treated paternalistically, with the presumption that they are 'too emotional to be able to decide' or without 'their whole decision-making capabilities because they are too stressed, for instance'" (Goering 2009, 10).

7 Researchers on gaslighting agree that an important feature of the phenomenon of gaslighting is that it can be done unintentionally. This raises substantive ethical and epistemological questions regarding the responsibility and accountability of the gaslighters.

8 On rape victims being disbelieved and the harmful consequences of this for their future lives, Whisnant (2017) writes:

> "Many rapes lead to additional harms beyond those intrinsic to the rape itself … Victims who do not reveal their rapes to others, whether due to shame or to the expectation that they will not be believed, experience profound isolation and lack of support; and indeed, many who do report their rapes are disbelieved or blamed by friends, family, and/or police. Due to both low reporting levels and low conviction rates, relatively few victims see their rapists punished; many of those raped by relatives, co-workers, friends, or other ongoing acquaintances must then face continuing interaction with the rapist, while those raped by strangers often fear that the rapist will find and re-victimize them."

9 Stories of early miscarriages make it clear that those women are made to feel ashamed in similar ways: mothers are not really allowed to grieve their early miscarriages, since the embryo is not considered developed enough to be called a baby, and many women are told that they should be grateful that the embryo did not develop into a baby that might have been "defective":

> "I found it really difficult to express just how difficult I was finding it emotionally after the miscarriage, and … I guess partly because I didn't know anyone else who'd miscarried and I felt sort of like, well, it was only six weeks. It wasn't like I'd lost … lost a baby or that I'd had a stillbirth or something like that … and you know that maybe I shouldn't be as upset as I was" (Leaney and Silver 1995, cited in McLeod 2002, 53).

10 This view does not necessarily lead to an infinite plurality of equally valid discourses. Various feminist epistemologists have discussed the difficult paths that must be followed in order to provide us with a plurality of discourses through the erosion of power structures without automatically consigning us to an absolute relativism; see Alcoff (2008); Code (1991); Code (2008); Harding (2008); Hartsock (1983).

11 Testimonial injustice is rampant in medical scenarios generally (Carel and Kidd 2014).

Women, though, are especially disbelieved. On the unjust lack of credibility women suffer within medical settings, see for instance Grundström et al. (2018); Reeves and Humphreys (2018).

12 Villarmea (2020; 2021) shows how the supposed irrationality, animality, and lack of control of female reproductive organs generally and the uterus in particular were used throughout enlightenment medicine and philosophy to justify women's general incapacity for rational thinking or reliable decisions.

13 The Facebook page "They Said to Me" features dozens of testimonies by women, mainly from the United Kingdom, who were systematically and pervasively distrusted in childbirth: "They said to me I wasn't having contractions would not believe me in 3 occasions sending me home with no examination, nothing. 4th time I could no longer tolerate the pain again I wasn't believed so I asked them put me on the baby monitor" ("They Said to Me" 2021).

14 Edwards's argument (following the more general argument of the body as a legitimate producer of knowledge and critiquing the mistaken belief that only a purely rational, disembodied mind can produce reliable knowledge) is enriched by phenomenological accounts presenting the embodied subject, or *lived body*, as itself producing meaning and knowledge. This challenges Cartesian understandings of the body as a simple "machine" at the disposal of consciousness, and of subjectivity and agency as residing mainly in the disembodied mind—understandings that reinforce dualistic models implying a passive body versus an active consciousness. Merleau-Ponty's (1995 [1945]) theory of embodiment as meaningful in its own right, as well as feminist phenomenological accounts (for instance Beauvoir's (1948) and Young's (1980)) of subjectivity as intimately embodied and ambiguous (constituted by both flesh and consciousness), provide rich possibilities for future exploration of the rejection, within medicalized labor, of the knowledge produced by the body and its fleshly experience.

15 Women's voices are more trusted in nonmedicalized childbirth settings. Jordan contrasts American medicalized childbirth with the midwife-led childbirth that occurs in the Netherlands: within less hierarchized childbirth scenarios, the woman (or the midwife, after consulting with the woman or

checking on her state) usually gives the cues for when to start pushing, for instance. There is no need then to "wait for the doctor," as Jordan puts it, since the birthing woman's voice is not systematically undervalued: "Midwives … by contrast, actively listened to the woman. Such listening is rare in most hospital settings because the staff's primary responsibility appears to be listening to and waiting for the doctor" (Jordan 1997, 75–76).

16 On unassisted births as strongly defying medical authority, a form of resistance to "bio-power," and on the stigmatization and persecution of the women who choose them by medical and legal institutions and society in general, see Miller (2012).

17 Other recent studies based on interviews with women postpartum (Hall, Whitman Foster, et al. 2018), as well as studies of plasma oxytocin levels coinciding with certain specific subjective childbirth experiences, strengthening the hypothesis that childbirth constitutes a psycho-socio-neurological event (Olza et al. 2020), equally suggest that women going through respected and undisturbed physiological labor experience fluctuating states of consciousness similar to those described in Dahan's work on the "birthing brain," and that they manage to labor more effectively in consequence. It is important to stress that Dahan's investigations constitute theoretical hypotheses and not empirical evidence. As she makes clear in her essay on the "birthing brain" (Dahan 2021a), the states of consciousness present in childbirth still constitute a neuroscientific lacuna since birthing women's brains have not been empirically investigated. Theoretical hypotheses about the brain states of birthing subjects and their recognition as part of women's efficient knowledge while laboring, however, urgently call for empirical research on consciousness during childbirth. If these hypotheses are confirmed, that could be very helpful in convincing medical staff that they should recognize, actively legitimize, and support these modified states of consciousness as productive and as providing "true knowledge" during labor. Even with the current lack of that particular empirical evidence, however, Dahan's studies (especially Dahan 2021a) do provide empirical evidence that the pregnant brain and the postpartum brain present multiple alterations coinciding with the state of "transient hypofrontality" and its already discussed features (such as diminished rationality and diminished inhibition), so that it would be at least reasonable to assume that during childbirth (the brief period between pregnancy and postpartum), the "birthing brain" most probably behaves similarly to the "pregnant brain" and the "postpartum brain" that immediately precede and follow it (rather than expecting those alterations to suddenly disappear during childbirth and reappear immediately afterwards).

3 #MeToo for the Labor Room

On Consent and the Opaqueness of Birthing Subjectivity

The feminist theorization of violence has worked on revealing the integral and essential masculine elements that structure and form our understandings of violence (Butler 2004; Butler 2009; Butler 2015; Butler 2016; Karhu 2016; Schott 2011), making it clear that many forms of gender violence are misrecognized or remain unseeable because they do not correspond to mainstream concepts of violence (Bergoffen 2012; Karhu 2016). Feminist theory has done much to broaden the spectrum of what is considered violence and illuminate how state violence is normalized or made invisible (Lokaneeta 2016), but much more needs to be done. Obstetric violence is still not fully acknowledged nor adequately articulated, whether by medical authorities or by birthing subjects themselves.

The epistemic problematic explored in this chapter concerns the capacity to identify particular obstetric practices as violent. My aim is not to explore differences in how obstetric violence affects various populations. Nevertheless, this analysis will show that class and race differences influence epistemic capacities, as obstetric systems reproduce racist and classist discrimination.

The Case of Vaginal Examinations

One constitutive feature of my own experience of obstetric violence was my constant subjection to vaginal examinations during labor. But I did not understand that then, nor even much later. I took it as just another painful "fact of nature" that doctors, residents, and midwives frequently inserted their hands into my vagina without asking permission, claiming that they needed to in order to understand why

DOI: 10.4324/9781003593829-4

I remained stuck for hours at eight centimeters dilation. It did not occur to me to question them or refuse.

As with many elements of obstetric violence, vaginal examinations during childbirth are mostly unquestioned, seen as a "natural," "normal" part of "labor management." Some laboring women experience vaginal examinations as intrusive and violent at the time, but many more—like myself—experience them as just another part of the blur of unquestionable, "typical" discomfort, pain, and shame in childbirth.

Many women lack the epistemic resources to recognize the practice of vaginal examinations during childbirth as violent, unnecessary, and potentially declinable. Throughout this chapter, I will note that this lack of recognition of and epistemic resources for understanding vaginal examinations as obstetric violence is the experience of many, but not all, women. I cannot claim that no women are equipped for such a recognition; some do experience these interventions as violent at the time, even resisting or refusing them—and this is how we know that these interventions are indeed violent. But this chapter addresses the reasons for the apparent underreporting and underrecognition, both by birthing women and by the medical community, of vaginal examinations in childbirth as violent interventions. Vaginal examinations during labor as currently performed in most medical settings are experienced as violent in some important sense; in a number of cases, they have been described as sexual or obstetric violence. Many reports of "birth rape" emphasize descriptions of vaginal examinations or other vaginal procedures (such as episiotomies), as we saw in the introduction: in her graphic narrative, Richland writes: "I was drugged and knocked unconscious. I was sexually assaulted: My vagina was cut and a man's tool (forceps) was inserted into my body" (Richland 2008, 43); and in the now-infamous "Kelly's Story," a terrifying case of "birth rape" was caught on camera in its entirety (Hayes-Klein 2014).

I am interested precisely in the massive silence and the inability to epistemically grasp the violence present in vaginal examinations, on the part both of very many women and, generally, of medical staff.[1] The analysis undertaken here, addressing epistemic hindrance and impeded recognition, precedes the question of consent: this analysis is necessary as a foundation, upon which any later analyses involving consent—our actual agency (or lack thereof) in granting or refusing to others our permission for them to act upon us—must then build.[2]

The specific case that vaginal examinations in childbirth go unrecognized as violence is part of the general problem that women ourselves frequently do not fully recognize obstetric violence. But vaginal examinations are even more clearly related to the sexual dimension of childbirth and the sexual self in general. A new discussion of the practice is needed, deploying the frameworks used to address sexual violence in addition to those that address the difficulty of considering benevolent medical scenarios as capable of featuring violence. That is what I undertake here.

Because it involves vaginal penetration, with all its surrounding sexual meanings, the violence in vaginal examinations is much more clearly related to sexuality than are other violent practices in labor (such as the Kristeller maneuver; physically restraining laboring women or forcing them to lie on their backs; verbal threats; or the denial of anesthesia or other medical help as retaliation when laboring women refuse to follow the medical staff's orders (Bohren et al. 2015; Silva et al. 2014)). This close relationship with sexuality, I argue, is precisely why the violence embedded in the performance of vaginal examinations during labor is so much more "invisible" and hard to conceptually grasp as violence. The difficulty lies not only in reframing systems (like the medical one) that are seen as essentially benevolent to understand them as capable of perpetrating violence, but also in framing sexual violence as violence in the first place. Even though in certain countries the Kristeller maneuver, say, is now recognized as a clearly violent obstetric practice, it appears that recognizing vaginal examinations as violent might take much longer. This will not change as long as sexual violence is not "framed"; as long as it goes unrecognized as violence; and as long as women's sexual availability and the existence of our bodies as shameful objects continue to be a normal part of our being-in-the-world.[3] There is an important distinction to be made among different kinds of obstetric violence. While all obstetric violence is gender violence, gender violence may take different forms—some involving physical control of women and verbal and physical disciplinary practices but less directly related to sexuality, and others, such as the violence in vaginal examinations, more clearly sexually laden. This distinction will be critical as we examine the epistemic mechanisms that prevent both laboring women and obstetrical staff from seeing the violence in obstetric violence.

Both sexual and obstetric violence have been normalized under oppressive patriarchal systems and frequently made unrecognizable, unseeable. In order for someone to fully recognize these as violence, they must first of all be named and reclaimed as such. This analysis is difficult to make because the argument relies precisely on silence, resulting from the lack of the epistemic resources women would need to fully recognize the practice's violence. Many laboring women never consider that they could question or refuse vaginal examinations. The practice is so normalized that it is not really seen as an intervention and hardly protested against. So then how do we know that this constitutes a violent practice? Many women do indeed bodily apprehend vaginal examinations as violent, but full epistemic recognition of this violence is obstructed, partly because the experience perfectly coincides with women's phenomenological situation within patriarchy and thus cannot really be framed as violent.

We must first examine this situation that renders sexual and obstetric violence invisible, nourishing the epistemic silence. A phenomenological analysis of women's embodied experience under patriarchy as always already essentially tied to sexual availability and commodification, and to shame, is crucial for explaining this epistemological impairment. I use a phenomenological take on Butler's (2009) distinction between "recognition" and "apprehension" to provide a more nuanced response to why vaginal examinations are not fully recognized and expressed as violent—even when they are, frequently, *apprehended* as such. Furthermore, Butler's ideas about the epistemic framings through which we make sense of different kinds of lives, as grievable versus ungrievable, help explain how the patriarchal sexual reification of women frames sexual violence as not-violence, ultimately preventing laboring women and obstetrical staff from recognizing vaginal examinations during labor as violence.

First, I present some existing investigations into the experience of vaginal examinations in labor, together with recent questions concerning their real benefits and how they might be considered part of a specific, medicalized understanding of childbirth and perhaps "a symptom of a cervical-centered birth culture" (Reed 2015). These examinations, frequently experienced by laboring women as painful, uncomfortable, and embarrassing, could in fact be greatly curtailed, even replaced. I then reflect on the lack of denunciations of this practice as violent, showing the silence to result not from laboring women's failure to apprehend its violence but from the epistemic deficiency deriving from women's situation under patriarchy and their phenomenological experiences within the context of sexual reification and shame. Finally, using Butler's framing of grievable and ungrievable lives, I offer a possible explanation for why both obstetrical staff and many laboring women are epistemically impeded from recognizing this practice—and, probably, obstetric violence more broadly—as violence. I end with reflections on a paradox that becomes evident in the course of this investigation: the reverse connection between privilege and the epistemic ability to recognize obstetric violence. This apparent paradox, however, resolves itself as not that paradoxical at all when we note that it makes sense that those who suffer most bluntly from obstetric violence sometimes would be best equipped for identifying it as such.

Vaginal Examinations during Labor: Desperately Seeking Women's Experience

Vaginal examinations in labor are mainly used to measure cervical dilation, in an attempt to assess the progress of labor. Several studies have pondered the practice's benefits and risks, the frequency with which it should be used, and how best to teach it to new midwives or obstetricians without unnecessarily harming women (Enkin et al. 2001; Hassan et al. 2012; Jha et al. 2010; Letic 2003; Roosevelt et al. 2018; WHO 2006). These studies have generally found that the practice is used much more frequently than medical evidence would recommend (Shepherd and Cheyne 2013; Stewart 2005). Discussions are currently taking place about how to perform the examinations in a way that is as respectful to and comfortable for laboring women as possible, and studies being developed on how to significantly reduce their use, even replacing them with less invasive practices (Hassan et al. 2012; Shepherd and Cheyne 2013; Stewart 2005).

It is important to recognize that vaginal examinations are not an indispensable part of labor: we can give birth without undergoing vaginal examinations at all. Laboring women should know that even for measuring progress in labor, vaginal exams are not the only, perhaps not even the most informative, option. Reed (2015) describes the practice as embedded in a "cervical-centered birth culture" that understands the laboring body as a predictable machine (see also Martin 1987) and makes a direct, unquestioning connection between cervical dilation and labor progress. Referring to Downe et al. (2013) and Ferrazzi et al. (2015), Reed reminds us that cervical dilation is not easily predictable or linear and that the evidence does not support routine vaginal examinations during labor. Vaginal examinations, she notes, belong to a specific, entrenched labor culture and are as hard to eliminate as many other practices belonging to the medicalized perspective on childbirth.[4]

Reed also discusses the disadvantages of vaginal examinations, arguing that they might be "inaccurate and misleading": again, unnecessary, and more about controlling the labor process than providing valuable information. They may also increase infection and/or result in rupture of the amniotic sac. But the most significant downside is probably the way in which many women experience the practice: as a painful, invasive process that may cause severe embarrassment, sometimes even PTSD (Dahlen et al. 2013, in Reed 2015). Yet we know little about women's experiences of vaginal examinations. The search for studies reporting such experiences unearths a considerable silence; very few such studies have been undertaken (Bonilla-Escobar et al. 2016; Bradby 1998; Broadmore et al. 1986; Hassan et al. 2012; Lewin et al. 2005; Ortega-Loubon et al. 2009; Swahnberg et al. 2011; Ying Lai and Levy 2002), and while this scarcity has been noticed (Bonilla-Escobar et al. 2016; Reed 2015), it has hardly been explained or theoretically tackled. This scarcity might be explained in part by clinicians' common reluctance to use patients' experiences as a central data point when evaluating the need to perform a given practice. Cook and Brunton argue that "clinicians' training requires them largely to discount patients' narratives in pursuit of the primary goal of a biological diagnosis" (Cook and Brunton 2015, 548, referring to Good 1994).

The paucity of studies is not, however, the main problem. In the present environment, even further studies might not reveal women's voices recounting their authentic experiences, their true apprehension of the vaginal examination. The experiences of laboring women in general—and concerning vaginal examinations in particular—are strongly linked to women's everyday experience in patriarchal society of deep sexual objectification and reification. Our bodies are experienced not as truly our own, as vehicles of our selves, but as alienated from our subjectivities. This experience of the body as fragmented, as not "in concert" with the self, is also tainted with profound shame (Bartky 1990; Young 1980). And this "normal" phenomenological experience of women under patriarchy precludes us from truly recognizing the invasive, even violent character of vaginal examinations, at least as currently performed in most medical scenarios—even though we may in fact apprehend the violence.

"The Water We Swim In": The Pervasiveness (and Invisibility) of Sexual Violence

In Cohen Shabot and Landry (2018), we note how feminist phenomenology is uniquely positioned to observe and deal with supposedly normal experience, which it presents as always already sexed and gendered. We analyze the #MeToo movement, showing how feminist phenomenology's insights into women's "normal" situation under patriarchy, embedded in sexual reification, shame, and sexual violence (including in Beauvoir 2011), continue to apply today—this is "the water we swim in": "That sexual objectification is just part of the humdrum of women's everyday lives reveals much about how women experience being-in-the-world" (Cohen Shabot and Landry 2018, 3). Reflecting on some of the #MeToo movement's viral texts, we show that sexual availability, passivity, and a continuous predisposition toward, or readiness for, discomfort, even pain, are the essential imprint of women's condition—even for presumed sexually liberated millennials. We cite Loofbourow's (2018) analysis of Roupenian (2017),[5] elaborating on why, in Roupenian's text, "consent" need not be the significant question at all. The #MeToo movement's greatest contribution to the discussion of sexual violence is probably showing that before there can be debate over consent, there has to be a discussion of the pervasive normalcy and thus invisibility of sexual violence. Women have learned not to see our own pain while becoming men's objects of pleasure[6]:

> Women have spent decades politely ignoring their own discomfort and pain to give men maximal pleasure. They've gamely pursued love and sexual fulfillment despite tearing and bleeding and other symptoms of "bad sex." They've worked in industries where their objectification and harassment was normalized, and chased love and sexual fulfillment despite painful conditions no one, especially not their doctors, took seriously … I wish we lived in a world that encouraged women to attend to their bodies' pain signals instead of powering through like endurance champs. It would be grand if women (and men) were taught to consider a woman's pain abnormal; better still if we understood a woman's discomfort to

> be reason enough to cut a man's pleasure short. But those aren't actually the lessons society teaches—no, not even to "entitled" millennials.
>
> (Loofbourow 2018, cited in Cohen Shabot and Landry 2018, 5)

Loofbourow's reflection can be directly imported into the discussion of obstetric violence and of vaginal examinations in childbirth in particular: discomfort, even pain, is women's normal experience of being-in-the-world. For black women it goes even further: their pain is not even considered normal but simply nonexistent. The racist idea that black women are less civilized, more animal-like (hooks 1997), and thus less likely to feel pain—that their bodies are more resistant than white women's bodies (Davis 2019)—makes black women even more prone to being quotidian victims of pain.

Shame

Women also experience their bodies under patriarchy as inherently shameful. This omnipresent shame allows structural mechanisms of violence and domination to obtain a strong grip on women and their bodies. Bartky (1990) argues that members of oppressed groups may experience a pervasive shame connected not with their own deeds but with their entire existence as objects for the other. This shame is paralyzing and unproductive, a direct consequence of inhabiting the world under a disciplinary gaze that requires bodies to persistently experience themselves as scrutinized objects (Bartky 1990, 97). Bartky's lucid analysis of pervasive shame and of women existing as permanent victims of shame belongs to a rich tradition of feminist phenomenological scholarship on female embodiment conceived under patriarchy as shameful, defective, in constant need of being tamed and rescued from itself (Beauvoir 2011; Cohen Shabot 2016; Dolezal 2015; Rich 1986; Young 1980; hooks 1997 [in the context of black women's bodies]; Lyerly 2006 [in the context of childbirth]). Dolezal (2015) writes:

> Women's bodies … are continuously positioned as inadequate or inferior when compared to these elusive body ideals; shame, and body shame in particular, becomes a permanent possibility … Women are already attuned to the feelings and contours of body shame; they expect their bodies to betray them and to deviate from

> the diffuse and invisible cultural standards of what a body "ought" to be. Failing to achieve the ideal body signals a deeper failed mastery of the body and corporeal control. This attunement to shame is so pervasive and indeterminate that it is often beyond the reach of reflective consciousness.
>
> (Dolezal 2015, 109–110)

On the normalization of obstetric interventions in childbirth and the cultural construction of the female body as defective, Vejlstrup (2017), a home midwife and birth activist, writes: "As long as the 'dangerous, sickly, female body' appears scarier to us than the vast number of serious injuries caused by labor interventions, patriarchy's medicalized imprisonment will falsely appear safer to childbearing women." In other words, patriarchal conceptions of women's bodies (often shared by women themselves) as inherently sick, weak, and polluted, are correlated with the assumption that medical interventions in childbirth—even violent and/or nonconsensual ones—are necessary. Thus, the epistemic obstacle to full recognition of the violence inherent in vaginal examinations in childbirth also involves women's essential shamefulness, the "dirtiness" of their bodies. Shame has been thoroughly investigated and pinpointed as one important mechanism for perpetuating obstetric violence by making it invisible: the "gendered shame" permeating women's existence allows for the hypermedicalization and unquestioned medical control of their "dirty" bodies. Obstetric violence is perpetuated because frequently, laboring women and their doctors see it not as violence at all but as the only way to "save" women from their overly sexual, polluted, shameful, untamed bodies (Cohen Shabot and Korem 2018).

Vaginal examinations may be the epitome of this taming of the polluted: the medical domestication of an inherently contaminated body. Stewart (2005) considers how vaginal examinations are "sanitized" by midwives who unnecessarily clean vaginas with various "hygienic" substances before or during vaginal examinations and use euphemisms when talking to women about their vaginas and these procedures. These examinations, Stewart argues, are a significant cause of embarrassment not only for birthing women but for the staff, who recognize this frequent, unquestioned part of the labor process as being very awkwardly intimate. Paradoxically, in attempting to "desexualize" the practice, they actually sexualize it by shaming and objectifying the vagina: refusing to name it, hiding it behind euphemisms, disconnecting it from a woman's embodied self (thus fragmenting her body), or even unnecessarily and literally sanitizing the examination, as if the vagina were truly polluted:

> The wash-down procedure described by midwives can be seen as a ritual to deal with their own discomfort about performing such an intimate examination. However, the fact that there was a wide range of practices suggests that the procedure is more than a means of dealing with embarrassment. Midwife F clearly perceived the woman's genitals to be dirty and in need of cleaning. The highly ritualized washing procedure she described and her use of a sterile pack mark the procedure as a professional event, and avoid any suggestions of a sexual encounter … However, such a performative wash-down can also be interpreted as an overt display of professional power and part of a disciplinary regime which aims to contain women's "leaky" bodies within a stable and controllable framework.
>
> (Stewart 2005, 591)

In what follows, I use Butler's (2009) framing of grievable and ungrievable lives to elucidate how this phenomenological normalcy of women existing as shameful sexual objects for themselves and for others—resulting in an epistemological blindness in, again, both women themselves and others—is produced and nourished by power, a political framing that marks lives as either livable or unlivable and thus distinguishes between what may and may not be legitimately recognized and named as violence.

Butler on (Politically) Framing Violence

Butler (2009) argues that in the context of war, certain losses are not mourned because they are never really considered lives to begin with:

> In targeting populations, war seeks to manage and form populations, distinguishing those lives to be preserved from those whose lives are dispensable … Ungrievable lives are those that cannot be lost, and cannot be destroyed, because they already inhabit a lost and destroyed zone; they are, ontologically, and from the start, already lost and destroyed, which means that when they are destroyed in war, nothing is destroyed. To destroy them actively might even

> seem like a kind of redundancy, or a way of simply ratifying a prior truth … Thus, there are "subjects" who are not quite recognizable as subjects, and there are "lives" that are not quite—or, indeed, are never—recognized as lives.
>
> (Butler 2009, 190–191, 198–200, 418–419)

Taylor (2018) uses Butler's framing to show how sexual violence against women is not truly recognized as violence, neither by the perpetrators nor, all too frequently, by the victims. She argues that because women's bodies are constructed in patriarchy as ambivalent—presumed to be both inviting sex (essentially available for others' sexual pleasure) and vulnerable, in need of constant surveillance—sexual violence against women is framed not as violence but as an expected, legitimate response to women's "nature," at least when the victim does not submit to strict gender regulations and rules of bodily scrutiny[7]:

> With respect to sexual violence against women, the normative distinction at stake is not so much whether sexual violence is morally acceptable or reprehensible, but rather whether sexual violence is or is not properly violence at all … If simply being embodied as a woman is "to ask for it," then any degree of male sexual attention directed at women cannot by definition be unwanted and, hence, a violation. This in turn calls into question whether such attention can be the sort of forcible and injurious action that constitutes violence.
>
> (Taylor 2018, 155)

Mardorossian (2014) provides another useful account of sexual violence, arguing that rape is only an extreme case, a particular form—not qualitatively different—of violence within patriarchy. All violence, she contends, is sexual, that is, gender-coded. The victim of violence (not necessarily or always a woman) is feminized, while the perpetrator occupies the masculine position. This economy of violence is so entrenched in patriarchy that—again—it becomes normalized and often invisible. The invisibility is enhanced within Western societies where there is an illusion that the law regulates violence, seen mainly as violence between individuals—not between the state or institutions and the individual. Mardorossian cites how rape is contested, resisted, and protested against in India, while in the United States the same phenomenon, of the same magnitude, is not protested as a phenomenon of social importance but seen as isolated, unfortunate cases of violence between individuals (Mardorossian 2014,11–12). It is not only sexual violence that is not framed, politically, as violence: medical violence—and specifically obstetric violence—is also difficult to frame, at least prima facie, as violence. This largely has to do with how violence is often conceptualized: as requiring intention, and as oxymoronic in spaces perceived as essentially benevolent or involving practices understood to be in the individual's best interest. Human childbirth is not a natural act; it is culturally constructed, and part of its medicalized construction is as a highly risky event where women need rescuing by medical authorities (Chadwick and Foster 2014; Katz Rothman 1982; Katz Rothman 2014). Therefore, defining what medical authorities do in childbirth as violence can seem puzzling, at the least.

Butler reminds us, however, that lives framed as "ungrievable," as "non-lives," (Butler 2009, 378) by particular operations of power are not really experienced as dispensable or valueless by those who live them. This remains true even when the attempt to recognize and formulate them as lives, or at least as lives that might be mourned when they are lost, is epistemically (or even ontologically) challenged. Butler formulates a distinction between "apprehension" and "recognition," apprehension being a much more elusive, less conceptual, more experiential—and, I would say, "embodied"—way of knowing than full recognition:

> "Recognition" is the stronger term, one that has been derived from Hegelian texts and subject to revisions and criticisms for many years. "Apprehension" is less precise, since it can imply marking, registering, acknowledging without full cognition. *If it is a form of knowing, it is bound up with sensing and perceiving, but in ways that are not always—or not yet—conceptual forms of knowledge.* What we are able to apprehend is surely facilitated by norms of recognition, but it would be a mistake to say that we are utterly limited by existing norms of recognition when we apprehend a life.
>
> (Butler 2009, 425–429; emphasis added)

Looking at obstetric violence in the light of Butler's explanation of the invisibility of sexual violence and Taylor's take on Butler's explanation, the question that arises is how women can epistemically frame this familiar, routine reality of violent obstetric practices as violence. How can women perceive obstetric violence as actual violence, rather than as a normal part of the "essentially benevolent" medicalized and medically managed childbirth process? Here, Butler's distinction between apprehension and recognition is helpful. Even when particular, politically loaded, frameworks forbid us from fully conceptualizing certain kinds of violence as violence, a more sensitive, perceptual knowledge is available to us as a way to know differently, to challenge and even shatter existing frameworks.

Butler does not elaborate much on what this "knowledge through apprehension" is like or how it is constituted, but phenomenological insights, particularly those resulting from feminist phenomenological analyses, can clarify the meaning of this distinction. Young (1980) explains how even though women's condition under patriarchy is one of profound objectification, women are never turned into absolute objects; a seed of subjectivity is always present. This also explains women's alienation from their own bodies: insofar as they perceive their own bodies as objects, women-as-subjects become alienated from those body-objects:

> The objectified bodily existence accounts for the self-consciousness of the feminine relation to her body and resulting distance she takes from her body. As human, she is a transcendence and subjectivity, and cannot live herself as mere bodily object. Thus, to the degree that she does live herself as mere body, she cannot be in unity with herself, but must take a distance from and exist in discontinuity with her body.
>
> (Young 1980, 154)

Thus, women apprehend their subjectivity even under extreme oppression and reification, even without any epistemological or ontological frameworks for recognizing or fully articulating this subjectivity. This is an embodied apprehension, through the lived body.

Clark (2018) quotes a doula who describes witnessing "birth rape" against one of her clients:

> The doctor walked in, put on gloves, and stuck both hands into the laboring mom's vagina. There was no consent. He didn't tell her he was going to do that or ask if she was okay with it. Moments later, he announced, "Oh, she is tearing already."
>
> *I had to look away because I could not physically handle what I was seeing. My body began shaking. I felt lightheaded; I felt*

> *frozen in place. [I felt] complete helplessness and fear and anger and grief.*
>
> I walked away from that feeling responsible in a way for what had happened, and knowing that this mom had just experienced something that shouldn't have happened, that something was really wrong. And that *there was this visceral response in my body to what I was seeing.*
>
> I just kind of remember being back in that place and feeling like there was nothing that I could do to change what was happening to this mom in that moment.
>
> *[I knew] my body was responding to something … even though I wasn't the person that it was happening to, I was still having this response and I needed to do something to work through it.* I knew I didn't want to be in that position again, feeling so helpless and frozen.
>
> (Clark 2018; emphasis added)

This description is illuminating because it presents the moment when the doula's "body speaks," even though she cannot, in that moment, articulate what is going wrong, or why, or how to respond. She can apprehend it, though: her horror is visceral. Her description perfectly exemplifies the "phenomenological apprehension of subjectivity notwithstanding oppression" that Young discusses.[8]

Vaginal Examinations as (Misrecognized) Sexual Violence—And the Paradox of Who Knows Best

Vaginal examinations in labor may constitute misrecognized sexual violence—often phenomenologically apprehended, but not epistemically recognized, as violence. Paradoxically, this lack of epistemic resources for fully identifying and possibly refuting the violence may be more pronounced among privileged women with access to advanced technologies and care than among marginalized, poor, or mistreated women, as there is, overall, a strong illusion of choice and of evidence-based care and treatment in wealthy Western hospitals and their maternity wards. Mardorossian, for instance, argues that the illusion of choice and of the medical institution's essential benevolence and nonviolence that prevailed in her own birth (and prevails within medicalized childbirth in the United States) prevented her, until much later, from seeing how violent her labor actually was (Mardorossian 2014, 87–89).

Birth experiences are deeply grounded in a concretely sexist, patriarchal reality and particular operations of power. This is crucial in explaining why certain populations are better suited to recognizing obstetric violence: where medical attention is already recognized as threatening and untrustworthy, obstetric violence is more easily recognizable as violence. In other words, laboring women who suffer blunt disrespect, poor medical care, and blatant verbal or physical violence may be more clearly able to articulate what is wrong with medicalized childbirth, and with vaginal examinations in particular. Previous childbirth experiences outside of obstetric wards and medicalized facilities—such as home births or midwife-attended labors—also provide women with a sharper perspective on what is or is not "normal," often allowing them to articulate how various obstetric practices might be wrong, sexually violent, or unnecessary and even giving them the power to refuse and resist those practices. Bradby (1998) gives an example of this in her study of rural Bolivian women's reactions to medicalized childbirth. The participants in Bradby's study, rural women who had migrated to the city, perfectly articulated how vaginal examinations performed within medicalized hospital labors unnecessarily sexualized their births, filling them with shame, fear, and anger. These women, who had previously experienced home births, where they were exclusively cared for by traditional midwives, understood and expressed that the frequent vaginal examinations they experienced as part of medicalized labor were unnecessarily painful, dangerous, embarrassing, and humiliating—and they often successfully resisted them. One woman explains: "I was in the Maternity Hospital and there were lots of medical students, and they were putting their hands up me a lot, and I said, 'Don't be poking me like that. I'm a person too. Do I look like a peasant woman for you to be poking me like that?'" (Bradby 1998, 53).

This paradoxical situation suggests that access to better epistemic resources does not always coincide with privilege and that marginalized populations suffering from lack of proper care, mistreatment, or even blunt violence may be more epistemically able to recognize this violence. This does not mean that they are better off—it just says something about how epistemic mechanisms develop. This definitely requires further exploration within investigations of the recognition of violence, in particular of obstetric violence.

I have discussed vaginal examinations during labor and the difficulties in framing them as violence. Many laboring women fail to conceptually and epistemically recognize them as violent. Women may, however, *apprehend* them as violent, and their embodied experiences may provide them with knowledge that could eventually be articulated and conceptualized, as we have seen here, for instance in the account of birth rape. The degree to which this is possible—resulting in full knowledge, but possibly leading to resistance as well—may also depend on the degree to which women are offered true choices, including exposure to alternatives to the medicalized model, in the form of home births or exclusively midwife-led births (Bradby 1998; Mardorossian 2014). The women in Bradby's study, for instance, had been exposed to alternatives to medicalized childbirth, which clearly affected their understanding of, sometimes even resistance to, hospital practices. Bradby concludes: "It is precisely because of this transitional state … where two cultural systems are in articulation with each other, that it is possible for women to articulate what for them becomes the extremely problematic nature of sexuality in childbirth. Their messages are clear and need to be taken into account in future policymaking" (Bradby 1998, 55).

A further question involves the obstetrical staff's ability to recognize these practices as violent. It is unclear how the staff, inserted into a political and cultural framework that fails to recognize sexual or medical violence as proper violence, might fully and responsibly recognize this violence and thereby become accountable for it. Until laboring women both recognize and speak up about the violence, others may not recognize it. Alas, the #MeToo movement has shown that even when women do raise their voices to denounce violence, powerful epistemic denial mechanisms nevertheless often prevent the recognition of that violence on the part of perpetrators.

An important difference between obstetric violence and sexual violence is that obstetric violence occurs *exclusively* within the hospital, one of the most essentially benevolent spaces we can imagine—and at the hands of people whose central role is to make us well. Sexual violence that takes place within insecure or violent contexts, on the other hand, is much more readily identifiable. However, the fact that sexual violence is often carried out within familiar or other seemingly "protected" contexts definitely blurs this difference.

There are two important points that need to be noted in this regard. The first involves the relation between privilege and epistemic power in the context of sexual and/or obstetric violence, which I have already described. As I noted above, the fact that less privileged women may, paradoxically, be better equipped to recognize obstetric violence requires further exploration. We can see it as an example of feminist standpoint theory, according to which the socially disadvantaged might in fact be epistemically privileged and the most capable of spotting oppressive patriarchal structures (Hartsock 1983). On the other hand, it represents a challenge to some recent scholarship on epistemic injustice, especially Fricker's (2007) notion of hermeneutical injustice, which contends that oppressed groups frequently lack the interpretive resources to comprehend and communicate meaningful aspects of their collective experience, implying that social privilege generally guarantees more epistemic power. Such concepts as "testimonial injustice" and "hermeneutical injustice" are useful for theorizing the epistemic difficulties involved in identifying obstetric violence: birthing persons are so oppressed and domesticated by institutions that they cannot recognize the violence they are treated with. But of course, as we have just seen, and in accordance with Hartsock, the opposite can also be true.

The second point I would like to develop involves the problem of consent in childbirth in relation to the subject's nonlinear, changing, ambiguous self. Anderson (2019) writes about this in the context of sexual ethics and sexual violence, emphasizing that consent is necessary but not sufficient for demarcating the true limits of a positive sexual experience: there is such a wide spectrum between "not being raped" and having a satisfactory sexual experience that the consent/non-consent binary is clearly inadequate for the complexity of sexual interactions. Anderson discusses many reasons why the concept of consent falls short: consent may develop into non-consent; consent presupposes "a proprietary notion of selfhood derived from social contract theory" and thus that "I can sign away my body"; heterosexual relations are constructed assuming that consent is almost always something for women to deliver and men to ask for; and "consent fails to register the temporally unfolding nature of sexual encounters." This is all relevant to the discussion of consent within medicalized childbirth and obstetric violence. However, what interests me the most here is that conceptualizing the subject as "relational"—constructed through interpersonal relations and thus never completely finished nor clearly delineated once and for all (a conceptualization I explored in chapter One)—contests the possibility of "clear consent," because such a subject changes during the experience itself and is never completely "transparent" to herself. This is Anderson's main theme, and it poses important questions regarding consent within childbirth. Anderson also suggests that consent is insufficient because "consent presumes a level of self-knowledge that individuals often lack. Many of us are often ignorant of our own desires, so suggesting that we can know what we want the moment we are asked overlooks historically coded forms of behavior, the effects of past experiences, and the relative power of differing social locations." This does not imply, however, that paternalistic protection should follow: in other words, that if we are ignorant of our own desires, maybe others know better what's best for us. Instead, it means that we need to develop more complex understandings of consent, taking into account a complex, dynamic self that is never crystal clear either to the subject herself or to those surrounding her:

> Within the context of sex, the idea that self-relation is not different in kind from relations to other beings does not give free license to paternalism, but rather suggests that we apply the same complex interpretive frameworks for negotiating our behavior with others to self-relations. Rather than taking my desires to be immediately transparent to myself, I might look at the ways they are revealed in various registers, including my behavior toward others and patterns of thought.
>
> (Anderson 2019)

These important insights into consent in sexual encounters may be key to rethinking consent in the birthing room: so far, obstetric violence has been discussed using a very straightforward notion of consent. But the experience of labor recalls that of a sexual encounter in several ways, and it seems vital not to oversimplify our understandings of consent in the labor room. Anderson's conclusion (in the context of sexual encounters) reveals much about what such a complexification of consent might achieve:

> In suggesting that we focus on the felt dimensions of our sexual subjectivity, I do not mean to suggest a turn to "raw" emotion at the expense of other dimensions of lived experience. The problem with the traditional view of consent is not that it overthinks sexual encounters, but rather that it underthinks the way that our feelings exist in relation to social scripts, relations of power, and the like. It presumes that people are rational agents with transparent desires

> that they may freely communicate to others. By conceptualizing sexual ethics on the basis of the heterogeneous self, we may better account for its complex intersubjective character. We may envision modes of self-fashioning that deepen our relations to others by recognizing that we are others to ourselves. This project takes us into still-uncharted territory, but I think it holds more promise than continuing to try building sexual ethics around a notion of selfhood inherited from social contract theory that feminist theory has proven wrong.
>
> (Anderson 2019)

Will such a complexification of consent also prove to be crucial and productive for the labor room? With this book, I try to provide resources for considering this and other urgent questions regarding the phenomenon of obstetric violence. From what we have seen in this chapter, however, it seems that a radical deconstruction of patriarchal values and medical hierarchies may be required in order for laboring women to truly be heard and for this kind of violence to be recognized and its eradication called for, finally, not only by its victims but also by its perpetrators.

Notes

1 For a more detailed analysis of birth rape and the feminist questions it raises, see Cohen Shabot (2016, 238–239, mainly footnote 9). There, vaginal manipulations were fully recognized as sexual violence. Here, however, as noted, I deal with the absence of recognition.

2 The notion of consent is itself problematic. On the specific case of gynecological examinations, see Cook and Brunton:

> "The Cartesian mind–body asymmetry in western medicine educates clinicians to privilege verbal consent, not to navigate contradictory "body talk" whereby bodies are legitimated as conveying needs contrary to those articulated . . . Ethical dangers include, for example, the ever-present possibility that consent will blur towards non-consent, with or without women voicing this shift. Another danger is that women may voice their assent but the clinician reads their body language as dissent" (Cook and Brunton 2015, 546–547).

Furthermore, the authors recognize the enormous difficulty of framing "consent" within asymmetrical power relations like those between doctors and patients.

3 Throughout this chapter, I deal with the idea that under patriarchy, women and their bodies are conceived as available for sexual exploitation and inherently shameful. There are significant differences in how nonwhite and white women's bodies are conceived in these contexts: both sexual availability and shame are also racially constructed. Black women's sexuality is much more often defined as promiscuous and lascivious than white women's sexuality, and shame and scorn are provoked and internalized according to these conceptions (Davis 2019; hooks 1997). For the sake of my argument, however, it is enough to recognize that sexual availability and shame are essential components of patriarchal conceptions of women and therefore importantly present in women's embodied experience within patriarchy, albeit in a variety of forms.

4 Reed reminds us that even women in less mainstream contexts have internalized this measurement culture. They, too, often want the "number," the "clear measure," to be confident of their progress—sometimes even when they truly understand that the duration of labor after a given measurement is very unpredictable.

5 Roupenian (2017) describes a typical, consensual heterosexual relation, insightfully revealing implicit violence and the objectification of women as our normal. Cohen Shabot and Landry write: "This is not a fictional piece on sexual harassment, on sexual assault, or on any other kind of extraordinary experience … To borrow from Beauvoir, this is simply women's 'situation.' Margot is reduced (women are reduced) to a body-object: hesitant and inhibited in her (our) intentionality. This curbing of our being-in-the-world as subjects of agency and action has the deleterious effect of causing us to forgo our own desires for the sake of those of others" (Cohen Shabot and Landry 2018, 4).

6 #MeToo thus appears to be relevant mainly to heteronormative framings of sex and sexuality. Queer theorists have criticized it for this reason. See Ison (2019); Rodriguez-Cayro (2017); Small (2018).

7 These gender norms are by definition impossible to satisfy; thus, even when the victim appears not to have "deserved" violence, sexual violence elicits no authentic surprise (Taylor 2018, 157).

8 The apprehension here of course belongs to a bystander rather than the laboring woman herself. La Chance Adams and Burcher (2014) develop the questions that this opens up about the power of solidarity, alliances, and intersubjective experience within labor and beyond; further research is also called for.

4 Making Ourselves into Objects

Complicity with Submission in Obstetric Violence

In the previous chapters, arguing that the phenomenon of obstetric violence needs to be recognized as a form of gender violence, I worked toward a conceptual and theoretical understanding of the different elements of the phenomenon. I have primarily addressed the violence imposed on women in complex and manipulative ways that they cannot resist, mainly because this violence is normalized, hidden by mechanisms of shame and various forms of epistemic injustice, and structurally embedded in how medicalized labors are constructed.

And yet, explaining what happened to me (and what happens to countless women in affluent contexts every day throughout the world) strictly in terms of imposed violence—as something of which we are nothing but passive victims, with no possibility of resistance through agency—would be doing a wrong to women for whom the experience of obstetric violence is the consequence of a reality of deep oppression, material scarcity, and utter discrimination. It would also mean turning a blind eye to the fine (or maybe not-so-fine) line that separates straightforward, inescapable, violent oppression from oppression that can in fact be resisted, even if only with difficulty—that difficulty being due to the strong internalization of the oppression, to the high price exacted from us if we do fight back, or even to an existential drive to *escape* freedom, to actively choose submission.

Thus, in this chapter I discuss the obstetric violence experienced by privileged women, like myself, as a phenomenon that requires at least a certain degree of complicity on the part of laboring women, of collaboration with our own submission.[1] This is a difficult position to be in. Seeing myself as a pure victim of evil is somehow comforting and reassuring: it obviously means that I need not think about responsibility

DOI: 10.4324/9781003593829-5

or whether I could have somehow resisted the violence. Nevertheless, I believe that a nuanced notion of our complicity with submission will add a valuable new dimension to the problem of obstetric violence, without necessarily engaging in "victim blaming." It will also be more equitable because it allows us to distinguish more accurately between my own experience of violent labor and that of women with no real alternatives whatsoever, those who are truly forced to succumb to violence.

In the following, I show how several analyses of privileged birthing women demonstrate the submission of these women to scripts of patriarchal femininity even before they are confronted with obstetric violence (that is, they could be said to have "facilitated" the violence, in a way, by willingly participating in their own objectification). All of the analyses, however, explain this submission by arguing that the women described have so profoundly internalized oppression and gender scripts that within their circumstances, their behavior is almost inevitable. But this blurs the differences between different kinds of oppression (that which is merely hard to resist versus that which is violently imposed) and, as I will show, cannot be a legitimate explanation of *complicity* with submission, given that complicity means precisely that we have not been forced, whether by external circumstances or internalized oppression, to submit. Complicity with one's own submission necessarily implies a certain measure of choice and freedom, a degree of agency, through which the subject *consents* to submit. I believe that we must develop an analysis that takes into account the possibility that at least certain forms of submission and objectification in the labor room are actively chosen—not just the result of internalized oppression or sheer violence perpetrated against birthing women—if we also want to grant these women at least a certain degree of agency and, more importantly, recognize in them a certain degree of power to resist objectification. To present a feminist phenomenological analysis of complicity with submission, I use Beauvoir's idea of "women's complicity with their own submission" as part of a more general phenomenological discussion of the subject of complicity with subordination, mainly as developed in Knowles's (2019; 2021; 2022) extensive work on this phenomenon. Knowles argues that a true discussion of complicity with subordination must address precisely the cases where we are driven to unfreedom without being actually forced to it (whether through actual violence or as a consequence of "adaptive preferences" or "internalized oppression").[2] Thus, complicity with subordination needs to be understood as something that happens when the subordinated one reinforces her subordination for reasons other than physical or emotional coercion: complicity requires agency (or it is not true complicity). In Knowles's comprehensive analysis, she uses phenomenology—mainly that of Beauvoir and Heidegger—to explain how the drive to escape freedom and turn ourselves into objects exists regardless of external sanctions or rewards. In Knowles's analysis, accomplices to their own subordination can be seen as having capacities for resistance and thus being at least partly responsible for their subordinated condition. I also argue that if it is true that phenomenologically, we are originally driven to unfreedom (and not naturally driven, in the absence of constraints, to choose freedom), then so are our bodies—meaning that it is not only patriarchy but also the original human tendency toward submission that pushes women to find solace in a silent, docile, domesticated body. No wonder, then, that women often actively wish to escape from the birthing body, which is paradigmatic of loudness, unruliness, and pollution.

Finally, I claim that if it is indeed possible for subjects who are not the victims of severe oppression to resist submission, then we must also judge it to be possible for many (privileged) women in the labor room, even if this resistance entails a supreme effort, in the course of which these subjects would abandon part of their known (embodied) identities and defy the inertia to submit to patriarchal scripts. But this resistance must also be supported and literally built, through demands that spaces where women give birth not be structurally constructed in such a way as to immediately push women to submit. In other words, we must demand responsibility not only from birthing women, but also (or mainly) from anyone surrounding them who might be in a position to help them resist the expected and quite understandable drive to submit, and who either does offer that help or refrains from doing so. I propose that one important way to create the possibility of resistance to oppressive practices in the labor room is to radically disrupt how the birthing experience, and within it the birthing body, are conceived by medical staff and by women themselves.

Obstetric Violence: Between Victimhood and Complicity with Submission

Today, most women around the world give birth in medicalized settings. Research shows that hospital births increase unnecessary medical interventions, failing to support physiological birth and frequently turning women's bodies into mechanical, mostly passive objects from which babies need to be delivered (Katz Rothman 2014; Martin 1987; Wagner 2001). Consequently, both hospital staff and birthing women have come to see births more as risky pathological events than as physiological ones—as dangerous, rather than normal embodied experiences.

I limit myself here to a discussion of obstetric violence as experienced by privileged women in relatively wealthy circumstances. In cases where the birthing woman is so marginalized and/or oppressed that resistance would mean death (when violence takes the pernicious form of deep oppression, scarcity of material resources, and lack of real, practical alternatives), the self-objectification of its victims is almost inevitable. In such cases, we cannot consider birthing women as accomplices in their own submission. As Garcia puts it, discussing women as dominated versus women who are accomplices of submission, the severely oppressed do not submit "in the sense that there is no real *will* to obey from the person who obeys, since the alternative is obedience or death" (Garcia 2021, 19; emphasis in the original).[3] On the other hand, the phenomenon that privileged women experience has proved to be less clear-cut and more complex (Behruzi et al. 2013; Smeenk and ten Have 2003; Wolf 2012); after all, what we are calling violence here is what many medical practitioners consider a normal scenario, one whose stated aim is to *benefit* women (usually in the form of a high degree of technological and medical intervention). Thus, since much of what the research considers violent is seen by medical staff as consensual practices performed on women as a result of real choices, the recent theoretical research on obstetric violence has been dedicated to critically evaluating and rethinking some of the concepts—including choice, consent, knowledge, and autonomy—that have been carelessly used within the discourse of birth (Dahan 2020; Malacrida and Boulton 2012; Chapters One and Three of this book). The main form of obstetric violence in this context appears to be dehumanization, i.e. turning women into birthing objects with no real agency, frequently achieved by the perpetration of various kinds of epistemic violence (Chapter Two).

The theoretical research on obstetric violence hypothesizes that one main cause for the phenomenon is the challenge that birthing bodies pose to patriarchal ideals of femininity. Birthing bodies are frequently active, expansive, and loud—prototypes of the phenomenological "I can." The patriarchal-medical powers, which cannot cope with an insubmissive femininity, a rebellious feminine body, therefore seek to "put them back in their place" (One). This is also one of the reasons why obstetric violence is considered a form of gender violence. But is this dehumanization and objectification of women carried out only by the medical staff attending the birthing woman? In the following, I show that birthing women themselves are also afraid of and threatened by this undisciplined, disruptive body: birthing bodies that are loud, raw, "dirty," and disobedient endanger women's identities as "feminine," as "proper women." Thus, women themselves often submit to the authority of the medical staff and dehumanize or "objectify" *themselves* in order not to transgress the rules of femininity, in order to return to femininity as quickly and securely as possible. And therefore, some women might be seen as cooperating, at least to some extent, with structural oppressive practices and with their own submission; they might be "turning themselves into objects" even before obstetric violence is actually performed on them. If this is true, then privileged women themselves might bear some responsibility for the perpetuation of the phenomenon of obstetric violence and for the possibility (even if limited) of resisting it.

Performing Femininity in Labor

Some investigations into how gender is performed in the birthing room provide good examples of the phenomenon of birthing women submitting to stereotypical feminine behavior in that context. Through countless accounts of privileged, middle class, heterosexual, mostly white American women performing birth in medical scenarios, Martin (2003) shows how birthing women willingly submit to disciplinary authority during their labor in order not to appear rebellious, nasty, or ungrateful. Sometimes, these women literally keep their birth from progressing in the way their physiology would dictate because they are too afraid of giving trouble, of being excessively loud or self-centered. Martin also shows that although some of the discourses of "natural birth" have permeated women's expectations of childbirth, "feminine" ideals demand a certain passivity even from women trying to birth naturally. Martin explains this phenomenon mainly through Foucault's (1979) and Gilligan's (1982) theories of the technologies of gender, discussing how women have internalized gender and the ways of performing it:

> These women tried to be polite, nice, and kind—to do the interaction work expected of them. Why? I argue that an internalized technology of gender caused them to be concerned about these matters. Such restrictions, feelings, and reluctance were a source of discipline and power over these women's birth experiences … I demonstrate that these women were often concerned with doing normative gender while birthing. They tried to do interaction work and to be nice, and they continued to attend to others' perceptions and feelings as much as or more than their own … When this gendered self breaks down, usually at the most difficult point of labor, women apologize for their deviant gender behaviors.
>
> (Martin 2003, 61)

Thus, the women Martin observes and writes about are afraid to stray from patriarchal rules of femininity even when their bodies are performing the prototype of a "feminine task," i.e., giving birth: it seems that the mere act of giving birth does not, in itself, constitute sufficient proof of femininity—kindness, care for others, and many other stereotypically feminine traits must also be maintained and exhibited, even in the moments during labor when the body is being extremely challenged. Here is one of the accounts cited by Martin:

> I remember between contractions here, I could hear the other people in the next room, and I remember thinking—'cause I was very loud at this point—and I remember thinking I felt bad because I was being so loud and this poor woman in the next room must be thinking awful thoughts about me. And then later the nurse came down and she said, oh, the person next door wants to make sure you were okay and if you had your baby, and so actually she was concerned and not angry that I disrupted her (Valerie).
>
> (Martin 2003, 62)

Martin's analysis, however, assumes that women are *compelled* to act this way—that is, that the rules of femininity are so absolutely and thoroughly internalized that women have no alternative but to submit to them. This, Martin hypothesizes, is why even in nonmedical scenarios, women will birth like good girls, so to speak: "Removing the medical institution from birth does not remove its social aspects nor make it natural and therefore free from male dominance … *Gender is in us, and we bring its power to discipline our bodies, selves, and lives to even the most natural events*" (Martin 2003, 70; emphasis added). According to this view, it would seem to be impossible to hold women (any women) responsible for renouncing their freedom—and thus, also, impossible to ascribe agency to women or demand resistance from them.

Further research appears to strengthen Martin's conclusions, since even though it seems that the birthing framework would make a difference, that difference proves to be only superficial. Carter (2009) shows that women birthing in nonmedical scenarios—whether at home or in midwife-led birthing centers—are more prone to deviate from stereotypical gender expectations, and not to apologize for it (in itself another such deviation). These women reveal a more potent embodied subjectivity, one that gives itself permission to deviate from passive, silent femininity without feeling guilty or ashamed. They oppose authority during their labor but, more importantly, they have already defied mainstream discourses on childbirth from the moment they chose not to give birth in a hospital. Carter hypothesizes, however, that the women in her sample have not completely abandoned gender expectations; that they are acting, instead, according to the rules of a femininity proper to the domestic realm, one that reflects a "good mother" (or good mother to-be) who is not occupied with obedience and submission to authority, as expected in a medical scenario, but is instead busy acting, being in control, and laboring as effectively as possible, even if that means being loud and improper:

> In the medical model, the definition of a good mother is likely to correspond with that of "good patient": one who accepts the idea that doctors and hospital staff are the experts at producing healthy childbirth outcomes and complies with their directions. Conversely, the midwives model of care contends that scientific research shows birth with minimal technological interventions is safest for babies, both physically and psychologically … In this context, birthing women may feel they must do whatever it takes to protect their babies from "harmful" medical procedures, even if it means behaving outside traditional notions of femininity. Viewed within this framework, participants in the current study appear to be defying smaller, everyday definitions of feminine behavior in order to achieve a larger, more significant feminine act. Thus, participants may be prioritizing different aspects of dominant definitions of femininity.
>
> (Carter 2009, 221)

Carter's and Martin's investigations both show, then, that middle class, privileged women, whether in medical or nonmedical scenarios, usually appear to birth like "good women": they either comply with medical authority, submit to its guidelines almost without protest, and keep their bodies as silent and constrained as possible, or else they perform a birth that is invested, in a different way, in domestic patriarchal conceptions of good motherhood.

More research shows that privileged women are also worried about preserving proper feminine embodiment during labor, trying to avoid producing too much dirt or mess. Thus, the "grotesque" body of childbirth—loud, expansive, and unruly—is frightening to, and rejected by, not only the medical staff but also birthing women themselves. Malacrida and Boulton (2012) produce multiple examples of (again mostly white, middle class) women whose choices in childbirth are dictated by the complex, sometimes contradictory heteronormative expectations of good motherhood, good femininity, and what patriarchy considers to be proper or ideal bodies and sexualities. These women try to negotiate the paradoxical demands of giving birth as "naturally" as possible, on the one hand, this being what "good women" and "selfless mothers" should aspire to, and, on the other, the requirement for their bodies to remain "clean," "tight," and, most importantly, sexually available for the male gaze and consumption. This research showed many women to be more preoccupied with embodying proper femininity during childbirth than with avoiding risks to their health. Caesarean sections were usually seen as inferior to vaginal births (from the point of view of how "selfless women" and "good mothers" should birth) but were also, at the same time, seen as a cleaner way to birth and as a better and, paradoxically, selfless option, but in this case with regards to effects on future sexuality. Vaginal births are "messy" and "dirty" and might, as such, be a real "turnoff" for men who have witnessed their partners giving birth, as well as leaving women vaginally "less fit" to satisfy their partners' sexual desires or demands:

> The interviews ... reflect the tensions women must navigate in relation to norms of feminine embodiment whereby women are expected to be demure and reserved, childlike and innocent, and birthing vaginally can be a violation/profaning of that purity and innocence. In particular, the unpleasant smells and sounds and the loss of fluids were cited as reasons vaginal birth is perceived to

> be messy, undignified, and degrading… . While vaginal birth is associated with a successful transition to selfless motherhood, it also conflicts with Western feminine norms that require women to be sexually selfless and remain tight, youthful, and constantly available for heterosexual pleasure… . Thus, ironically for some of these women, having a Caesarean birth was constructed as a selfless way to maintain their prepregnancy bodies and thus remain sexually receptive and attractive to their male partners.
>
> (Malacrida and Boulton 2012, 768)

Malacrida and Boulton, like Martin and Carter before them (and like other studies in this vein, including Dixon-Woods et al. 2006 and Malacrida 2015), interpret these results as proof of the irresistible oppression in the contradictory cultural requirements of femininity that are irremediably internalized by wealthy women giving birth. But even if this does indeed constitute an important part of the story of women in the medicalized labor room, I believe that another layer needs to be added to these interpretations, especially when dealing with privileged women birthing in wealthy contexts—women who are not crushed by racism, precarity, or utter violence and do not appear to be the helpless victims of oppressive surroundings (although they are influenced by dominant patriarchal ideals), but who in fact enjoy power and agency in many aspects of their lives and frequently resist and offer alternatives to various patriarchal mandates. Thus, in the following, I discuss the issue of complicity with submission, arguing that the women portrayed in these studies cannot be seen simply as victims of internalized patriarchal ideals, without agency or any possibility of resistance. It is not that the argument that gender norms are internalized is wrong, but that that is not all there is. I wish to complicate the argument by discussing how some women actively choose to become objects, to escape freedom, even when they do not necessarily have to and even when they are conscious that they might have alternatives.

In other words, even when certain ideals of femininity are clearly acting on women, we must nevertheless recognize a measure of complicity and self-objectification in the cases described above, particularly if we want to be able to distinguish between the condition of these women and that of utterly oppressed ones, and if we want to understand and imagine forms of resistance and change as emerging from women themselves. This might also provide new lenses through which to view obstetric violence—as a phenomenon that might sometimes take place in a scenario that is already "polluted," one where women willingly make themselves into objects even before the specific structural violence of the birthing room reaches them.

A Phenomenology of Women's Complicity with Their Own Submission

> One can only talk about submission when there is no active resistance to power, when the attitude or the action expresses *a will of the agent*. Submission is thus, at a minimum, the result of *a will* to not actively resist domination.
>
> (Manon Garcia, "We Are Not Born Submissive"; emphasis added)

Feminist philosophy has found it painful to explore the phenomenon of complicity with one's own oppression, or submission to an unfree existence. The reasons are evident: drawing attention to how women might in certain cases be complicit with their own submission and thus at least somewhat responsible for it, or expected to resist it, could be seen as a kind of backlash, a form of victim blaming, or as threatening to obfuscate women's most urgent problem under patriarchy: the true violence toward and domination of women. I believe, however, that discussing this issue can in fact strengthen the feminist struggle, since clarity and an increase in epistemic resources generally prove to provide more possibilities for liberation and resistance.

Beauvoir discussed this phenomenon seriously and comprehensively, mainly in *The Second Sex* but also elsewhere. She called for responsibility and action from bourgeois women like herself, frequently portraying them as subjects with the capacity to recognize and embrace their own ambiguity, their existence as both immanent and transcendent—as subjects who could resist objectification but decided not to: they *chose* to escape ambiguity and made themselves into objects, in part because this was easier and provided them with material and other benefits. Women's complicity with their own submission, in such cases, thus does not derive exclusively from internalized oppression—it is, rather, the result of a choice that was made:

> In the upper classes, women are *willing accomplices* to their masters because they stand to profit from the benefits they are guaranteed. We have seen that women of the high bourgeoisie and aristocracy … do not hesitate to radically sacrifice their autonomy as human beings; they stifle all thinking, all critical judgment, all spontaneity; they parrot conventional wisdom, they identify with the ideal imposed on them by the male code; in their hearts, and even on their faces, all sincerity is dead.
>
> (Beauvoir 2011, 663; emphasis added)

Beauvoir thus firmly distinguishes between two groups of women: on the one hand, women who are so deeply objectified and lacking in resources (sometimes even the resources with which to imagine a different situation), that it would be an ethical mistake to hold them responsible for their condition, because freedom, even as a possibility, is almost completely unavailable to them; and, on the other hand, those who have a choice but actively choose submission and, because they have a choice, also bear at least some responsibility for choosing one path rather than another. This is a crucial point in Beauvoir's theory of freedom, because she clearly proposes freedom as situated: in Beauvoir's view, some people and groups of people are freer than others, and thus more responsible than others. Oppression is always a matter of degree, and so is the possibility of resistance. Beauvoir already states this very clearly in her earlier *Ethics of Ambiguity* (1948):

> It is then that we discover the difference which distinguishes them from an actual child: the child's situation is imposed upon him, whereas the woman (I mean the western woman of today) *chooses* it or at least *consents to it*. Ignorance and error are facts as inescapable as prison walls. The negro slave of the eighteenth century, the Mohammedan woman enclosed in a harem have no instrument, be it in thought or by astonishment or anger, which permits them to attack the civilization which oppresses them. Their behavior is defined and can be judged only within this given situation, and it is possible that in this situation, limited like every human situation, they realize a perfect assertion of their freedom. But *once there appears a possibility of liberation, it is resignation of freedom not to exploit the possibility*, a resignation which implies dishonesty and which is a positive fault.
>
> (Beauvoir 1948, 38; emphasis added)

Beauvoir thus argues that certain women choose or consent to become objects, to become unfree. (On Beauvoir's apparently colonialist and ethnocentric assumptions here, see Altman 2020.)[4] Beauvoir clearly does not consider these women to be living in total "ignorance" or "error"—otherwise they would be like slaves, or like women trapped in an oppression so violently imposed that escaping it is either unimaginable or would require the sacrifice of their very life.[5] The woman who "resigns" freedom, according to Beauvoir, is the emancipated woman who, due to narcissism[6] or a fear of losing privileges and benefits, remains passive, sticking to her condition as object as a part of the patriarchal prescriptions for femininity. This is further complicated by the fact that complicity with our own submission corresponds to our original existential condition: we are born into a ready-made world that we consider normal and necessary. Such is the child's condition that Beauvoir describes in the quotation above. The tendency to escape, to turn away from freedom, because of the anxiety that uncertainty and ambiguity cause us, is, thus, what originally characterizes us as humans—and not, as Knowles claims, exclusively a product of imposed oppression: "On a phenomenological account, then, the imposition-independent dimensions of complicity are explained in terms of our attempt to avoid ambiguity and uncertainty and renege self-responsibility" (Knowles 2022, 12).[7] Thus, choosing freedom is a moral imperative (and in fact an achievement) precisely because it is not the automatic or first option available.

This anxiety and tendency to escape from freedom are even more pressing for women, because they are constructed as objects in patriarchy. Kruks uses Beauvoirian categories to explain the complicity with submission that Beauvoir (2011) describes in several parts of *The Second Sex*: the phenomenon is a response to a woman's understandable need to reach congruence and avoid ambiguity, a way "both to resolve the painful paradox of being a subject whom men posit as a thing and, simultaneously, to evade the ontological ambiguity of embodied subjectivity by positively identifying themselves with their objectification" (Kruks 2012, 72). In other words, for Beauvoir, women's complicity with their own submission constitutes a rational, congruent choice, mainly in that it coincides with what women have learned that their social self is, and is expected to be.[8] This is also what Garcia argues in her analysis of Beauvoir's idea of submission. Garcia amplifies Kruks's explanation, emphasizing the embodied dimension of the phenomenon of complicity with submission as it occurs among women in patriarchy and arguing that Beauvoir recognizes the congruity—and even *pleasure*—that being objectified entails for a woman: being seen as a beautiful, sexual object disambiguates a woman's embodied existence, turning her into the object of consumption that she is expected to be (Garcia 2021, 156). However, these are explanations, not justifications, for such behavior. Beauvoir appears to consider women's complicity with their own submission to be consistent with patriarchal expectations of them, but nevertheless morally reprehensible (when our situation of privilege allows for resistance) and something we ought to insist on fighting against. Women's complicity with their own submission thus appears to be a version of bad faith, albeit a less pernicious and thus less morally troubling version: in actual bad faith, we are confronted with our true self, which threatens us with its absolute, overwhelming freedom, and we decide to escape its burden (McWeeny 2016). But escaping freedom because of the anxiety that knowing ourselves to be originally, truly free causes us—as the concept of bad faith proposes—is not the kind of complicity with submission that Beauvoir is referring to. A woman's complicity with her own submission is not what happens to someone who fears her "original" absolute, overwhelming freedom but rather what happens to someone for whom submission constitutes the core of her social identity—her *situation*, to use Beauvoir's concept—and for whom rebelling against that submission thus threatens to destroy her, almost to abolish her own self as she knows it.[9]

Thus, even if a woman is to be considered at least partly responsible for this self-objectification, she should not bear the same responsibility that a privileged man should bear for choosing to escape his own ontological freedom in an act of bad faith: choosing freedom does not constitute the kind of threat to a man's identity and place in the social world that it does for a woman, who is socially constructed as an object.

Adaptive Preferences, Complicity with Submission, and Responsibility

One of the most comprehensive and compelling analyses of complicity with subordination is the analysis developed by Knowles (2019; 2021; 2022). Knowles relies on Beauvoir's and Heidegger's phenomenological discussions of complicity with submission, or chosen unfreedom or subordination, to emphasize how such complicity must be understood as being active, and as performed with agency, if we really want to regard it as complicity. Complicity derived from internalized oppression or adaptive preferences (that is, derived from inclinations emerging as a necessary result of imposed oppression) cannot be taken as true complicity. In opposition to those who theorize submission as only being possible as the result of external or internalized oppression, Knowles insists that both Beauvoir and Heidegger recognize the human tendency to choose self-objectification and to reinforce and embrace submission—and escape responsibility—even when conditions in fact allow for freedom:

> The approach from adaptive preference assumes that what *really* needs to be explained is what and how external factors can impose things on us in such a way that we turn away from our own flourishing and become complicit in our own subordination. A phenomenological approach rejects the natural trajectory claim and takes complicity as a baseline. In this respect, complicity is not a response or reaction to external circumstances, as it is for the adaptive preference theorist. It is not primarily imposed, nor is complicity some kind of defect ... What the phenomenological analysis I have developed highlights, therefore, is that even if nothing was imposed upon us, self-responsibility might still be refused, and thus, an agent could still be complicit in their own subordination.
>
> (Knowles 2022, 9, 12; emphasis in the original)

Knowles thus recognizes what she calls "personal complicity" (with subordination) as the phenomenon in which we are both the perpetrators and the victims of oppression. In such a case, it is not an injustice or a wrong, as it is when we participate in oppressing others. However, these boundaries blur because our personal consent to submit frequently helps to perpetuate the oppression of others like us; for instance, "the woman who believes that what other people call 'sexual harassment' is a necessary part of courtship" not only "helps to perpetuate a world in which her freedom is limited as a result of sexual harassment" but also helps to reduce the chances that women who are sexually harassed will be heard, and even that they will be able to conceptualize their own experience as one of harassment (Knowles 2021, 228).

Thus, responsibility needs to be taken when freedom and agency are a possibility, not only for our own sakes but in order to participate in the construction of a freer and more just world for others. Even when we are not the direct creators of the situation that constrains our freedom, if we are not compelled to submit and we can envision another possible scenario, we are responsible for resisting our own oppression and even for acting in such a way as to bring about liberation:

> We find ourselves complicit not through our own actions, but because of the circumstances and ways of Being into which we are thrown. But this responsibility becomes less vicarious and more "owned" when we fail to ready ourselves for the possibility that things could be different, and refuse to take responsibility for our complicity. This failure to respond to our situation by continuing to unquestioningly take up the world as it is presented to us is something for which we must hold agents responsible if there is any hope of bringing about change.
>
> (Knowles 2021, 236)

Conclusions

To illustrate the phenomenon of privileged women who become complicit with their own subordination, Knowles (2019) presents an analysis of the backlash to the #MeToo movement, specifically the backlash from privileged women. In Knowles's eyes, such an

> acceptance of sexual harassment and the "resignation" to a world in which it is just part of everyday life … is a flight from the possibility of resistance and manifests … [an] active complicity in accepting and helping to perpetuate the idea of women as sexual objects, an understanding of women that limits their social and material freedom and suppresses their possibility to express and live in light of their existential freedom.
>
> (Knowles 2019, 257–258)

In the same vein, I argue that for many privileged women—women who, like myself, have not been obviously forced to give birth in medicalized settings (nor clearly compelled to submit to certain practices or to violence)—it is complicity, not just oppression, that helps to perpetuate unnecessary interventions in labor and other forms of obstetric violence. Thus, when laboring women silence themselves; when they ask to remain immobile and to be controlled by the medical staff, wanting the staff to make decisions for them; or when they begin the birth process primarily wishing their bodies to remain "clean," tight, sexually available—then we must recognize complicity with oppressive practices and with submission. The loud, active, disruptive birthing body constitutes a threat not only to the medical staff but also to the laboring woman herself, who may well fear losing the benefits of remaining objectified in labor (which include the possibility of total reliance on medical authorities, achieving a "clean" and "sterile" birth that is completely managed by other people, and freeing the woman from the pangs of responsibility). Moreover, women are frequently so appalled by the rebellious agency of their bodies and their embodied selves during labor that they flee those bodies and selves, actively choosing submission instead. (On the birthing body as rebellious and "unfeminine," see also the introduction to this book.)

The oppressive structure that sustains medical birth—its use of epistemic violence, and of sanctions when women do not comply—is clearly the major force behind the dehumanization of women in childbirth. In the arguments above, however, I have shown that it is not the only such force. In the previous chapters, I discussed obstetric violence as an oppressive practice of which women are mostly victims. And yet a neat and simple approach that discusses obstetric violence exclusively through the perpetrator/victim binary cannot explain it in its totality. It is undeniable that many women are seduced by the benefits of a submissive labor and phenomenologically driven to be silenced or to choose (unnecessary) medical intervention, even to comply with violence—even before it has been forced upon them. Thus, I hope that there is illumination to be found in a more nuanced reading, one dedicated to understanding why privileged women frequently submit to, and comply with, unnecessary, even violent, practices in the labor room. New feminist discussions of submission, such as the ones I have dealt with in this chapter, help us understand that women agree to submit not only because the cost of resisting is too great but also because even in the absence of constraints, we are not automatically driven towards freedom: we are, in fact, frequently phenomenologically pulled to submit and to choose our own objectification.

For a woman to rebel against submission is to contradict her situation in patriarchy and thus the social expectations to which she is subject—it goes against her core identity. There are therefore not many or obvious good reasons to choose rebellion. Within the frameworks of existentialism and phenomenology, however, freedom is always a possibility, which means that there is a call to take responsibility. While our compliant identity is indeed deeply entrenched in our embodied selves, and it is not at all easy to give up, "this does not mean that complicity is inevitable or something from which we cannot pull away" (Knowles 2022, 13).

This is not at all to say that privileged birthing women bear the sole or even the main responsibility for their own objectification and dehumanization in labor. These women might facilitate that process by embracing their own submission and objectification, but those in power—i.e., the medical staff and all who are in charge of the medicalized birth (and of perpetuating its dehumanizing structure)—are in a position, within the event of birth, of much more privilege than that possessed by even the most privileged birthing woman, and thus bear the main responsibility for avoiding the alienation and dehumanization of women in childbirth. Even though this analysis has highlighted the phenomenon of women's complicity with their own submission in childbirth, it is imperative to recognize that in spite of the natural tendency of women within patriarchy to submit, or maybe precisely *because of* that tendency, the medical staff, in turn, has the responsibility to actively draw laboring women away from their own understandable and congruent propensity to objectify themselves as an expected and normal part of the birth experience (and of women's situation in patriarchy in general).

Nevertheless, as I have laid out here, a change in the structure of medicalized childbirth by itself is not enough to end the violence against women in the labor room. The phenomenon of women's complicity with their own submission must also be attended to.

Notes

1 Garcia explains why she deals specifically with the problem of submission as it regards privileged Western women—why this is a more problematic and philosophically interesting discussion:

> "The greater women's freedom of choice, the more problematic their submission appears. The moral issues this book is focusing on appear when submission is not the result of clear coercion but appears as a choice. In this respect, focusing the analysis on the societies in which women and men are at least formally equal—that is to say, they have the same legal rights, overall—allows me to examine submission in its most morally complex forms" (Garcia 2021, 14)

This does not mean that unprivileged women cannot be accomplices in their own submission—it is just that in their case, there are many more evident conditions reinforcing their submission, primarily their *actual oppressive situation*, the imposed oppression and violence that come from without.

Throughout this chapter, I use "complicity with submission," "complicity with subordination," "complicity with oppression," "chosen unfreedom," and "self-objectification" interchangeably. All of these formulations appear within the literature pointing to the same phenomenon; or, at any rate, the subtle differences among the concepts they describe are not significant to my argument. They all refer to an active negation or renunciation on our part of our own existence as free subjects, a self-objectification and an active complicity in our own submission to others' authority.

2 For a compelling account of the phenomenon of "internalized oppression" or "adaptive preferences" and the difference between this phenomenon and that of "complicity with submission," see Knowles (2021a). Knowles defines adaptive preferences as

> "…preferences formed in response to oppression, which serve to uphold or reinforce the oppressive social structures that are imposed on the agent as a result of their situation … Adaptive preferences are commonly presented as unconscious adaptations … They are often thought to be the result of lifelong habituation … Some argue that adaptive preferences are 'paradigmatically non-autonomous' … while others deny that non-autonomy is definitional for adaptive preferences and draw attention to conscious and rational adaptations, which can nevertheless be seen as adaptive because they reflect the situations of oppression in which they were formed. What unites this diversity of accounts is the idea that adaptive preferences are in some way imposed on the bearer as a result of their situation of oppression" (Knowles 2021a, 2–3).

I deal with this in greater detail in the following.

3 Whether or not this implies that deeply oppressed people are absolutely deprived of agency is a complex question, one that the existentialists (especially Beauvoir, in the particular context of deeply oppressed women) dealt with constantly in their work. Agency appears to be a matter of degree, seen as deeply affected by material and situational constraints, for most existentialists (although less so for Sartre, who considered freedom never to be truly meaningfully bounded by our situation). I deal with this in more detail in the following. Here, it is enough to recognize that women affected by obstetric violence in precarious contexts are not to be made responsible for not resisting forceful, life-threatening violence. This does not mean that they are absolutely unable to imagine their situation as different or to think of alternatives—just that when they do not, they are not to be blamed or made responsible for it. On Beauvoir's and Heidegger's view of freedom and situation as importantly different from that of Sartre, Knowles writes:

> "The understanding of how our situation and our relations with others can influence our possibilities, and our possibility for freedom at an existential level, is an insight that Beauvoir and Heidegger share. But it

> is an insight that is unavailable to the Sartre of *Being and Nothingness*, who argues that our situation can never truly limit our freedom; insisting that it is instead 'our freedom which constitutes the limits which it will subsequently encounter' (Sartre 1943/2003, 504)" (Knowles 2019, 7).

For more on different types of consciousness under oppression, see McWeeny (2016).

4 Altman (2020) extensively discusses this passage and the various reactions and criticisms its seemingly colonialist or ethnocentric assumptions have elicited. Altman argues that rather than blaming Beauvoir for being patronizing, in this case toward Muslim women, we should read the passage as Beauvoir's way of distinguishing between those who should at least be held responsible for their own unfreedom and those whom it is much less possible, if at all, to hold responsible:

> "The opposition here is not between western and 'Eastern' women, or between modern women and some group of women that have been left behind; the opposition is between those who are able to free themselves and those who aren't, and there are some of these in each (geographical and temporal) category … Beauvoir's use of 'the woman in a harem' is a way of arguing that all situations are not alike and that not all subjects are practically free, even though theoretical freedom may be the heart of what it means to be human. Without the understanding that situations are different, and that situations matter, no understanding of oppression, indeed no politics at all, is possible" (Altman 2020, 223; 376–377).

5 Knowles challenges the interpretation that Beauvoir's argument simply means that Beauvoir sees privileged women's complicity with their own submission as just a product of internalized oppression, which can never be truly resisted:

> "It is not simply that women accept their position as the Other because they have no other option. Indeed, if they did this would not, strictly speaking, be a case of complicity. Complicity implies the ability to do otherwise. I cannot be complicit in something I cannot avoid doing. The unfreedom of complicity is not simply something that is imposed from without, as is the case with most instances of oppression. Rather, as we see elsewhere in *The Second Sex*, the unfreedom of complicity is something that is embraced from within" (Knowles 2019, 5).

6 Melo Lopes uses Bauer's analysis of the narcissist in Beauvoir to provide an extensive, compelling account of Beauvoir's concept of narcissism and its relevance for explaining complicity with submission: "For Beauvoir … the narcissist is someone who regards herself in a deeply incoherent way: as primarily a passive object that she herself—as an active subject—can glorify. In actively striving to become an exalted object, she demonstrates precisely that she is not one" (Melo Lopes 2021, 708). I will not deal specifically with

the discussion of the narcissist here; that is beyond the scope of this paper, and there are other concepts regarding complicity and submission that are more relevant to women's complicity with submission in the particular context of the labor room.

7 In Heideggerian terms, we can say that *Dasein* is originally and constantly seduced to fall into *das Man*, thus renouncing freedom and responsibility. Knowles writes:

> "Through its stubbornness Dasein turns away from its existential freedom by taking the social roles and dominant narratives prescribed by *das Man* to be definitive of its own existence, essentially binding on it, and thus unchallengeable. Being stubborn with regard to the social roles and narratives in terms of which Dasein currently understand[s] itself can thus be interpreted as a central way in which Dasein flees the burden of its own existence and becomes complicit in its own unfreedom" (Knowles 2019, 14).

Therefore, Knowles argues, "the phenomenological analysis implies that complicity is the starting point of all agents" (Knowles 2022, 230; see also Knowles 2021, 11).

8 Knowles explains this in similar terms, comparing Beauvoir's metaphysical stand on the human condition with Heidegger's:

> "Returning to Beauvoir's metaphysical understanding of human existence, we can view woman's stubbornness and resignation as an attempt to resolve the ambiguity of her existence by reifying it in terms of a fixed social position or dominant social narrative. For Beauvoir, as for Heidegger, attitudes of stubbornness and resignation can be understood as a central way in which active complicity manifests itself" (Knowles 2019, 15).

9 Knowles (2019) turns to Heidegger to explain the difference between his and Beauvoir's understandings of complicity with submission, on the one hand, and Sartrean "bad faith," on the other:

> "Heidegger's account of falling into *das Man* is not analogous to the Sartrean notion of bad faith. It is not an account of the artificial obstacles we put in our own way, obstacles that can never really constrain us or limit our freedom. Rather, Heidegger's account of *das Man* speaks to the way oppressive social settings can play a central role in restricting our self-understandings and what we believe we are capable of, thereby limiting our possibilities for existence and suppressing our existential freedom" (Knowles 2019, 8).

For more on the difference between bad faith and the Beauvoirian idea of "making ourselves objects," characteristic of women's consciousness under patriarchal conditions of oppression, see McWeeny (2016).

5 Conclusions

Keeping Birthing Bodies Grotesque—Or Reclaiming Disorientation

Where Do We Go from Here?

Throughout this book, I have shown that feminist perspectives on how and why obstetric violence happens occupy a central place in the recent research on the subject. What is still missing from the research, however, and still demands to be studied is the link between the female body (especially the female birthing body) as grotesque and monstrous, on the one hand, and obstetric violence as a tool for domesticating and "cleaning" that body, on the other. Looking at the birthing body and the phenomenon of obstetric violence through the lenses of theories of the grotesque (themselves connected to theories of dirt, disgust, the abject, and the monstrous) and crip phenomenologies (which discuss disability, disorientation, and abnormality as "emancipatory spaces," rather than spaces to be avoided or escaped from) will allow us to illuminate how obstetric violence is understood and even offer new practical ways to tackle it.

The use of disability theories (and within them crip phenomenologies) to discuss bodies that are not typically disabled has raised some concerns about the problem of appropriation: can and/or should these theories be used by nondisabled people, and can their deployment to discuss experiences not exclusively pertaining to the disabled be justified, either morally or intellectually (Steele 2023; Young 1997)? However, many scholars working on such theories (including those I cite here) see the field as highly intersectional and the lines separating abled from disabled bodies as frequently blurred, suggesting that this theoretical frame and methodology might rightly be used to illuminate experiences lived by the nondisabled as well (see for instance Schalk 2017a, b). Thus, here I use disability theories (mainly in the form of

DOI: 10.4324/9781003593829-6

crip phenomenologies) in their broader meaning: as a resource for studying and discussing not only typically disabled bodies but other nonconforming bodies as well—bodies that rebel against normativity and thus constitute a challenge to hegemonic powers (and are therefore frequently sanctioned or oppressed by those powers). Garland-Thomson's "broad understanding of disability," which is central to her concept of "feminist disability theory" as "radical critique," considers disability a "pervasive cultural system that stigmatizes certain kinds of bodily variation … [and] has the potential to incite a critical politics" (Garland-Thomson 2020a, 185). I base my proposal here on this comprehensive idea of disability, and of disability theories in general and crip phenomenologies in particular as constituting a "radical critique," one that is strongly related to queer theory in the broad sense, as Warner, for instance, understands it: "a politics directed against shame and normalization, and aiming at a complex mobilization of people beyond sexual identity" (Warner 2012, 2). But this proposal for future research, as I will show, also attempts to provide resources for better understanding the obstetric violence that is indeed exercised toward disabled bodies, gender nonconforming bodies, and bodies laboring with "nonproductive" labors—such as those that result in a dead fetus or baby.

What Kind of Violence Is Obstetric Violence?

As I have previously discussed in this book, feminist phenomenology and feminist epistemology have been used to try to disentangle the mechanisms that nurture and enable obstetric violence in the form of practices that seem normal, necessary, or inevitable—both in the eyes of medical staff and, more pressingly, even in those of birthing women themselves (see Chapters Two and Three). Feminist phenomenology has contributed to showing how the birthing body is a rebellious, subversive body, a prototype of the "I can," a potent embodied subjectivity, and one that frequently behaves in ways considered unfeminine according to patriarchal standards because of the power, strength, loudness, and expansiveness that it displays. Obstetric violence, thus, has appeared as the tool through which these bodies are "put back in their place": through obstetric violence, the subversive body that is characteristic of labor is dominated, silenced, restricted (Chapter One). In other words, it is "made feminine" again—sometimes through severe violence, even reported as torture (Cohen Shabot and Sadler 2023).

Phenomenology and the Birthing Body as "Abnormal"—What Does Obstetric Violence Have to Do with It?

Laboring bodies, however, are not just strong, loud, powerful bodies: they are also vulnerable bodies in need of solidarity and care (though not in the form of paternalistic impositions; Chapter One). They are also bodies that belong to the "abnormal" due to their changing form and capacities: they are unexpected, sometimes disoriented, ambiguous bodies that can be suggestive of monstrosity. Birthing subjects are irremediably, clearly embodied and their embodiment is fleshy, smelly, and replete with fluids, "dirt," or "contamination" (frequently including feces and urine and always including blood); as such, they are surrounded by shame and fear (Cohen Shabot and Korem 2018; Lyerly 2006; Stewart 2005). One of the most illuminating studies of birth as "dirty" is Callaghan's (2007), which explains the history of birth as a "dirty zone," along with the social, political, and cultural functions (both past and present) that are served by defining birth that way: the strengthening of the power of the medical establishment and its absolute control over birth. The medical establishment, Callaghan shows, has deemed birth dirty mainly so that that establishment can be the one to "sanitize" it—to take on the primary responsibility for making it hygienic (while an important part of the history is that, at least in its beginnings, this medical attempt to "sanitize" birth actually increased infections and deaths). The medical system also displaced midwives from the birth scene by declaring them, too, to be dirty. In short, Callaghan argues, what is behind the need to "cleanse" birth is power relations: diminishing the power of midwives and—even more critically—that of the laboring woman. Unlike Callaghan, I do not think we need to affirm that birth is not "really" dirty in order to question the compulsive need to "clean" and "sanitize" birthing bodies. My assumption is that birth is indeed grotesque, dirty, and monstrous—but not threatening, dangerous, or in need of control and sanitization, except when looked at through the normalizing perspectives of patriarchy and medicalization.

Birthing bodies are thus prototypes of Kristeva's (1982) "abject," and therefore frequently escaped from, both by the medical staff and by laboring women themselves, because they are grotesque bodies in need of being cleaned, sanitized, and "saved" from their own monstrosity. I have already cited Vejlstrup (2017) on the normalization of this attitude: "As long as the 'dangerous, sickly, female body' appears scarier to us than the vast number of serious injuries caused by labour interventions, patriarchy's medicalized imprisonment will falsely appear safer to childbearing women" (see Chapter Three). This scary body is a prototype of the "uncanny"—it is deeply familiar, intimate, and yet strange, dangerous, and anxiety-inducing. The idea of the uncanny has been widely used in recent philosophical studies on health and disease, mainly to stress the anxiety provoked by the paradoxical condition of the ill body, experienced as being simultaneously profoundly close (to the self) and alien, unknown (Aho 2020; Trigg 2020). The birthing body presents these features too, as I discuss below.

Thus, I argue, obstetric violence cannot be thoroughly understood without addressing the grotesqueness of laboring bodies, their inherent uncanniness and unexpectedness, and the challenge that all of this poses to the ambitions toward standardization, normalcy, order, cleanliness, and predictability that are paradigmatic of medicalization (Bost 2005; Liese et al. 2021; Zorzanelli et al. 2014). A new phenomenological analysis examining these features of birthing bodies is much needed in order to add a different perspective to the research on the causes behind the phenomenon of obstetric violence. A crip phenomenology—one that challenges the conceptions of "normal/abnormal" and "abled/disabled" bodies and places—will create space for a novel discussion of obstetric violence and the strategies for tackling it.

The "Abnormal" Birthing Body as a Grotesque, Subversive Body

Although birthing bodies are not abnormal in the sense that they perform a rather normal, physiological function, they are abnormal compared to what is expected from normal bodies in everyday life. Birthing bodies are grotesque bodies: they change form; they are fluid, expansive, and both comic and monstrous.[1] Their openings are exaggerated and dynamic; they are bodies that go out and into the world and that receive or meet the world through their orifices. Bakhtin describes grotesque embodiment precisely in this way:

> The grotesque body is not separated from the rest of the world. It is not a closed, completed unit; it is unfinished, outgrows itself, transgresses its own limits. The stress is laid on those parts of the body that are open to the outside world, that is, the parts through which the world enters the body or emerges from it, or through which the body itself goes out to meet the world. This means that the emphasis is on the apertures or the convexities, or on various ramifications and offshoots: the open mouth, the genital organs, the breasts, the phallus, the potbelly, the nose. The body discloses its essence as a principle of growth which exceeds its own limits only in copulation, pregnancy, childbirth, the throes of death, eating, drinking and defecation. This is the ever unfinished, ever creating body.
>
> (Bakhtin 1965, 26)

Grotesque bodies are disruptive bodies par excellence, subversive bodies that challenge the norm, though not always through strength or extraordinary capacities. Frequently, in fact, it is through the opposite. They are hybrid bodies that often include deformations that create disabilities, such as limbs and body parts that are too big or too small, disproportional and thus dysfunctional, or that present a mixture of incompatible embodied features. I will use different theories of the grotesque body as transgressive (Harpham 1982; Kayser 1963; but mainly Bakhtin 1965) to inform a novel analysis of the birthing body as challenging medical discipline and power, not by being an extraordinarily potent, abled body but in its character as a nonnormative crip entity. This novel analysis should allow us to understand the phenomenon of obstetric violence in a new light: as the very predictable response of the medicalized system to the unbearable anxiety caused by the dysfunctionality, disorientation, contamination, challenge to binarity, and lack of control that grotesque birthing bodies entail.

Crip Phenomenology: Embracing Disorientation

> More loudly and more forcefully, *we need to talk about the worlds disability creates.*
>
> (Joel Michael Reynolds, *The Life Worth Living*)

> The main function of others as toeholds is not to interact with us in ways that reorient us, so much as to meet us in ways that make disorientations livable.
>
> (Ami Harbin, *Disorientation and Moral Life*)

Within the field of disability studies, crip phenomenology has emerged as a form of critical phenomenology[2] that looks at the experiences of disabled bodies and subjects and of people living with physical or/and mental illnesses.[3] This new phenomenological research does not aim to recognize these bodies as pertaining to some new normal—to expand the notion of normalcy in order to include all bodies by bringing them to the same table[4]—but rather to emphasize dysfunctionality, sometimes even presented as a kind of monstrosity. The purpose is to argue for the disabled body and the disabled subject as possessing certain virtues and to analyze disability as a condition from which new insights into experience and the lived world might emerge. Bringing crip phenomenology to the fore can contribute to the depathologization of the birthing body and promote a reading through which it can be approached as an "emancipatory space" (Sandberg 2018, in Foth and Leibing 2022), instead. One of the main goals of crip phenomenology has been to embrace disorientation (Harbin 2012; Harbin 2014; Harbin 2016)—to argue for the (ethical, aesthetic, and epistemic) value of being lost, of encountering others in the midst of confusion and uncertainty.[5] I shall argue that such an attitude toward the lived experience and the lived world might aid in resisting obstetric violence: a medical system that (even partially, even critically) adopts the idea of disorientation as a space in which it is possible to linger, and that incorporates other important reflections on the potential of illness offered by crip phenomenology, might thereby become better equipped to deal with the grotesque birthing body and less prone to attempt to tame or control it through violence. This attitude could also help birthing subjects to embrace their own disoriented birthing body, instead of fearing it and thereby becoming complicit in their own submission to medical objectification (see Chapter Four).

I believe that the introduction of insights from crip phenomenologies into the field of birth studies might open up myriad new ways of looking at what happens in medicalized birth settings as a consequence of fear and anxiety in face of the unexpected, the disorienting, the grotesque, and the monstrous. This could also offer an important approach to questions regarding trans men and gender nonconforming subjects giving birth (as well as disabled laboring bodies), for whom the descriptions of grotesqueness and monstrosity might apply even more strongly than for more mainstream birthing bodies (Garland-Thomson 1996; Nirta 2021; Zigarovich 2018). Obstetric violence toward disabled subjects, trans men, and other gender nonconforming subjects giving birth has not been investigated. This research would present an invaluable opportunity to approach this pressing issue, mainly through the insights provided by crip phenomenologies. Another phenomenon that is worth investigating through this prism is that of obstetric violence toward laboring subjects when the fetus is no longer alive, that is, people experiencing late miscarriages or undergoing abortions (Bellhouse at al. 2018; Ravaldi et al. 2018). The presence of a dead fetus, I hypothesize, redoubles the monstrosity and grotesque character of birth: it adds to its liminality and uncanniness and may be responsible for producing even more shame, anxiety, and loathing on the part of both the medical staff and the birthing subjects themselves. The attempt to control this may in turn provoke even more blatant violence.

But how exactly does the birthing body constitute a grotesque body? How are violence and the need to domesticate the birthing body related to this body being paradigmatic of monstrosity and disorientation? How, precisely, is it the vulnerability of this body, expressed through its tendency to be broadly open to the world, polluted, and replete with uncontrollable fluids and dirt—rather than this body's potency and strength, as I have argued before—that provokes obstetric violence?

The Grotesque Female Body

> ALL HUMAN SOCIETIES have a conception of the monstrous feminine, of what it is about woman that is shocking, terrifying, horrific, abject.
>
> (Barbara Creed, "Horror and the Monstrous-Feminine")

The grotesqueness and "abnormality" of the female body have already been discussed by grotesque theorists (Bakhtin 1965; Kayser 1963; Kuryluk 1987; Russo 1995) and at length by several feminist scholars: women's bodies have been recognized as paradigmatic of fluidity, viscosity, blurred and leaky limits and boundaries, porosity, contamination, and liminality in general (Braidotti 1994; Cohen Shabot 2008; Creed 1986; Creed 2015; Creed 2016; Douglas 1966; Kristeva 1982; Shildrick 1996; Shildrick 2015). Women's bodies are thus surrounded by shame (Bartky 1990; Dolezal 2015).

In addition to being grotesque, female bodies have also been recognized as monstrous. In her classic essay on the monstrous body and its place in posthumanism, Shildrick describes the female body as a "broken," disruptive body that threatens the masculine subject and is responsible for provoking anxiety by being a "transgressive signifier" that challenges the norm and the normal: "women are the non-subject other, the excluded, the embodied, the monstrous … Women's bodies, paradigmatically, and by elision, women themselves, exemplify an indifference to limits evidenced by such everyday occurrences as menstruation, pregnancy, lactation and such supposedly characteristic disorders as hysteria. Women are out of control, uncontained, unpredictable, leaky: they are, in short, monstrous" (Shildrick 1996, 1, 3). Some feminist studies of reproduction and reproductive (in) justice have discussed the monstrosity of female embodiment as critical for understanding the various wrongs committed against women in medicalized systems dealing with reproductive issues—including in pregnancy and postpartum (Huet 1993; Tyner 2023; Ussher 2006). However, the specific event of birth has not been thematized, even in works, such as Ussher (2006), that extensively address women's reproductive bodies and monstrosity. Thus, detailed research into the grotesqueness of the birthing body and the birthing process is still very much missing. A specific focus on birth is necessary and will provide new and original insights because the birthing body is a doubly grotesque body: on the one hand, it is grotesque simply by being female, but in addition, the body acting in birth is replete with grotesqueness even if we set aside its female character.[6]

In order to discuss the birthing body as compatible with grotesqueness and monstrosity, I rely on the vast literature that has demonstrated the laboring subject to be one in which fragmentation, fluidity, excessiveness, confusion, irrationality, dirt, uncanniness, and undecidability rule. Various studies on the experience of birth show the birthing body as possessing these qualities, and they also show how difficult it is for the medical system, even sometimes for birthing women themselves, to properly cope with and react to this embodied experience without shame, without a need to control this body and to manage and articulate the experience and the body of birth, and without resorting to a clear, rational, unified, and unambiguous idea of the subject (Cohen Shabot 2020; Edwards 2005; Jordan 1997). It is imperative to stress that grotesqueness and monstrosity in themselves do not necessarily imply shamefulness: grotesque and monstrous bodies are shameful, dangerous, anxiety-provoking only when looked at from the perspective of "normalcy" as a value (as happens within patriarchy and frequently within medicalization). Thus, it can be value-neutral or even positive to define birthing bodies as grotesque and monstrous, if a "normalizing" perspective is not taken as the basis—if we challenge the idea that grotesqueness and monstrosity are synonymous with danger and must be regulated.[7]

Recent studies specifically dealing with disabled birthing bodies are also of great relevance (Hall, Hundley, et al. 2018; Redshaw et al. 2013). I rely here to a great degree on Chadwick's (2009) illuminating study of birth experiences as paradigmatic of uncontained subjectivity, in which the women who attempt to articulate them nevertheless end up resorting to a classic, unified subjectivity. Chadwick's qualitative research shows how a certain methodological tool—in this case a Kristevan theoretical framework, one that emphasizes a non-unified self as the basis of experience—is useful when trying to more accurately bring to the fore specific aspects of certain birth narratives. These narratives, Chadwick argues, frequently present elements that exceed "normal" narrative framings, but the women telling their stories nevertheless continue to use those framings in order to attempt to control the birth experience, to contain it within the limits of, for instance, clockwork time and unified subjectivity. But Chadwick clearly shows that, with adequate methodology, the body is able to penetrate the barriers of language and present itself in all its irrationality and excessiveness through the birth narrative, even if only for moments.

I believe that the radical, excessive, disruptive character of the birth experience can indeed be narrated given the proper methodological tools and framings. In the case just cited, Chadwick makes use of a Kristevan paradigm. We can significantly broaden our ability to talk about the birth experience in a different manner and thus also to understand it, socially, culturally, politically, and even medically, in a different manner, by approaching it through the paradigm of a crip phenomenology. Chadwick's conclusions are also important for how they emphasize the potential of this novel understanding of childbirth to affect "phallocentric, individualist and modernist conceptions of the self" (Chadwick 2009, 130). Further contributions to this philosophical endeavor will provide further insights into how a different understanding of the birthing experience and the birthing body might also make significant changes to our conceptions of experience, embodiment, and subjectivity, even outside the particular context of birth.

Another important body of work that presents the birthing embodied subject as exceeding rationality—as disoriented and "disordered" (and succeeding precisely because of these qualities)—is Dahan's (2020; 2021a; 2021b; 2021c) research on what she calls "birthing consciousness." Dahan hypothesizes that what allows birthing bodies to labor effectively is precisely the irrationality of the "birthing brain," since, according to empirical evidence, women achieve a state during undisturbed physiological birth that suggests "transient hypofrontality," a brain state similar to those present during the use of certain drugs, hypnosis, or deep meditation. Because of the reduced neocortical activity, this state of consciousness is characterized by a lower level of rationality—it presents more disinhibition, but far from being detrimental to birthing women, this less rational state of consciousness allows for a more physiologically effective birth. Dahan's research, I propose, supports my argument on the birthing body as needing to be understood as a grotesque body: an excessive, disoriented, irrational, and changing body that the medicalized system feels required to control and contain.

Once we accept the birthing body as excessive, grotesque, and even monstrous and therefore provoking feelings of shame, powerlessness, and helplessness in medical staff and in birthing women themselves,[8] it is possible to argue for the use of insights from crip phenomenologies in order to embrace this grotesque birthing body, to understand it on its own terms instead of trying to change and control it. Crip phenomenologists—mainly following the work of phenomenologists such as Heidegger (1962; 1993) and Merleau-Ponty (1964; 1968; 1995 [1945])[9] and heavily influenced by the work of Butler (2016) and other queer theorists (including Halberstam and Halberstam 2005; Halberstam 2011; Warner 2012), as well as theorists advocating for a deconstruction of the myth of the unified self and the healthy body as the ultimate human goal (Murphy 2011)—have presented physical and mental illnesses as productive, emancipatory spaces from which we can learn to aesthetically appreciate the estrangement and uncanniness, the "misfitness" that is characteristic of our existential condition (Carel 2007; Carel 2016a; Carel 2016b)[10]: we are never at home in the world; unpredictability and randomness rule; and in our search for security we construct fictitious entities such as a unified self and an ordered life, attempting to make of our future an expected one.[11] Crip phenomenologists take the estrangement brought about by illness as an opportunity: instead of trying to "cure" illness and abnormality, to smooth them over, they look at their epistemic and aesthetic emancipatory potential. They see illness and the disorientation within it as paradigmatic of the general uncanniness of the existential condition: "The possibility of losing one's grip on home anchors the constitutive role of un-homelikeness, estrangement, contingency, and unpredictability in human experience. My suggestion is that these elements are important for our understanding of disorientation in illness" (Lajoie 2019a, 555).

Far from trying to "cure" disorientation or normalize our lost subjectivities, then, crip phenomenologies suggest that these features are precisely what sustains human relations: the intersubjective relations of care and mutual protection necessarily derive from the recognition of vulnerability and disorientation, even if they clearly do not constitute the only response to those, given that people also respond to disorientation and uncanniness with oppression and violence meant to abolish those uncomfortable states. However, we can argue in favor of an ethical responsibility to respond to disorientation with compassion (Lajoie 2019a).

Thus, I propose that we should think of creating not spaces in which birthing bodies (women's and others') will be oriented, but rather spaces that will be "supportive of the experience and expression of such disorientations" (Lajoie 2019a, 561). Looking at the disorientation that is characteristic of laboring bodies, and viewing the experience of birth, with awe[12] instead of with fear and repulsion, might, I argue, bring about significant changes in how the medicalized system and birthing women relate to birth, hopefully contributing to a consciousness-raising about both obstetric violence and the complicity of birthing women in their own submission, as well as about why and how to resist both of those phenomena.

Notes

1 Grotesqueness does not equal monstrosity (not all the grotesque is monstrous, and not all monstrosity is grotesque), but birthing bodies are both grotesque and monstrous: the features of the grotesque body are clearly present in birthing bodies and birthing bodies are monstrous at least by virtue of being female or "other" (not cis male), as I discuss in the following.

2 While classic phenomenology reflects on lived experience by reducing it to its basic transcendental structures and attempting to elucidate the intimate relation between the subject and its world without looking at specific contexts and influences, critical phenomenology both develops from and challenges classic phenomenology, emphasizing how "contingent historical and social structures also shape our experience, not just empirically or

in a piecemeal fashion, but in what we might call a quasi-transcendental way" (Guenther 2020, 12). Thus, critical phenomenology takes seriously the different forms in which our particular situations shape our experience. Crip phenomenology is a subset of critical phenomenology, specifically dealing with experiences of disorientation and "misfitness" due to disability and/or illness—experiences that other nonnormative bodies and situations also frequently encounter.

3 Reynolds (2022) distinguishes between disability and illness, developing an illuminating critique of what he calls "the ableist conflation"—the common medical and philosophical conflation of disability with illness, pain, and suffering (thus defining a disabled life as necessarily involving suffering and therefore, according to normative conceptions of "a life worth living," falling short). This important distinction does *not* imply that the lives of people who have illnesses that *do* involve pain and suffering are a priori worthless. I use the insights provided by Reynolds and others into the lives of disabled subjects and the lives of those living with illness—they all have a place within crip phenomenologies and are relevant, I argue, for the discussion of the birthing body.

4 As Mia Mingus (2011) writes about the disabled subject: "We don't want to simply join the ranks of the privileged; we want to dismantle those ranks and the systems that maintain them" (in Lajoie 2019a, 561).

5 The idea of disorientation, which occupies a central place within crip phenomenology, raises important questions about the reinforcement of "the normal," by way of disorientation's own definition as that which misses the "right" path. As I will show, crip phenomenologies see disorientation as a matter of degree: it is part of the existential condition in general, but it is more or less strongly present depending on the specific situation or experience we inhabit. Illness, for instance, invites a large degree of disorientation. Thus, evidently, the construction of "the normal" is more oriented toward certain bodies, objects, and situations than others (Ahmed 2006). The question of whether "the normal" should be changed in order to provoke less disorientation, or whether disorientation should be maintained and embraced as a cardinal part of our existential condition (even by reinforcing the present "normal"), is one that meets with diverse and ambiguous responses within crip phenomenologies and that poses important philosophical challenges.

6 I believe that the proposed research can also be the basis for deep research on trans and gender nonconforming birthing people. Trans people are considered even more monstrous than women (Nirta 2021; Zigarovich 2018), and birthing redoubles their monstrosity. If the freakishness of birthing women can be explored and redeemed through crip phenomenology, that research might help to construct a safe space for other birthing people as well. For an analysis of trans pregnancy, see Drouillard (2021).

7 Many of the scholars dealing with grotesqueness and with monstrosity emphasize their positive role as resources for challenging social and cultural norms, offering subversive modes of thinking, and bringing about social change (Bakhtin 1965; Cohen 2007; Russo 1995; Shildrick 1996).

8 Many women are afraid of and disgusted by their own birthing bodies (see Chapter Four). The subject of pain in childbirth is also relevant to discussions of the birthing body as excessive and as provoking feelings of shame and impotence in birthing persons and the medical staff, its special character, and how it wrongly triggers the usual medical responses to pain: namely the need to control, mitigate, cure, and abolish that pain—responses that many birthing women themselves also embrace, but that are inadequate to the complex realm of labor pain (Cohen Shabot 2017a; Cohen Shabot 2022b; Dahan 2019). Reynolds's (2022) extensive and illuminating discussion of pain from the perspective of critical phenomenology as well as Kolářová's (2010) discussion on negotiating disability and pain through queer S/M practices are also illuminating in this context.

9 For an interesting commentary on the relevance of Heidegger (1993) for explaining the anxiety and uncertainty experienced during the pandemic, see Aho (2020); see also Cohen Shabot (2022a). For an extensive and illuminating discussion of Merleau-Ponty's relevance to disability studies, see Weiss (2015). Merleau-Ponty's concept of "one's own body" (1968; 1995 [1945]) (*le corps propre*) is shown to be relevant to issues surrounding grotesque bodies mainly because it is connected to ideas of what is considered clean and "appropriate"—as well as to questions of agency and the limits of the embodied self. Merleau-Ponty's "body proper" attempts to draw a clear line between one's own embodied self and the body of the other: "The break between my body (the body proper) and the body of the other separates two irreducible forms of bodily experience" (Stawarska 2006, 101). But Merleau-Ponty's body proper is always "cracked" anyway, and thus discontinuous and ambiguous in itself. This is precisely what allows intercorporeality: "The concept of intercorporeality is thus deeply ambiguous: on the one hand it suggests continuity between myself and the other, an absence of definite boundaries, but this continuity is made possible only because of a sense of *discontinuity*, estrangement, anonymity, even dispossession, that prevents my body from ever being unambiguously my own" (Marratto 2020, 198; emphasis in the original).

10 "Misfitness," coined by Garland-Thomson (2011; 2020b), has become one of the main concepts within disability studies, mainly referring to disability as a constant possibility for all embodied subjects and as a relational category, always dependent on the material and social conditions surrounding bodies.

11 Crip phenomenology has continuously and rapidly evolved, mainly during the last decade, discussing and deconstructing central philosophical themes

such as the nature of the self, time, and space and asking existential and political questions about what should be expected from life (how the "life worth living" (Reynolds 2022) should be defined and recognized), while pointing to the oppressive and heteronormative basis of the prevailing definitions of physical and mental health and of the "proper" body and the "proper" way to approach disability—thus challenging dominant paradigms of medicalization in important ways. This is not an exhaustive list of the researchers discussing these issues (and some of them fall not strictly into the category of crip phenomenology researchers but rather into the broader field of disability studies and queer theories of illness), but all of the following inform the present analysis and might significantly enrich any further research on the subject: Abrams (2016); Foth and Leibing (2022); Hall (2021); Harbin (2012); Harbin (2014); Harbin (2016); Kafer (2013); Lajoie (2019a); Lajoie (2019b); Lajoie (2021); Lajoie and Douglas (2020); McRuer (2006); Reynolds (2018); Reynolds (2019); Reynolds (2022); Sandberg and Marshall (2017); Steinborn and Nusbaum (2019); St. Pierre (2015).

12 On the experience of birth as one that potentially produces awe, and on the epistemic possibilities of this awe, see Dahan (2023).

References

Abrams, Thomas. 2016. "Disability, Queer Phenomenology, and the Politics of Personhood." *InterAlia* 11: 1–18.

Abramson, Kate. 2014. "Turning Up the Lights on Gaslighting." *Philosophical Perspectives* 28: 1–30.

Ahmed, Sara. 2006. "Orientations: Toward a Queer Phenomenology." *GLQ: A Journal of Lesbian and Gay Studies* 12 (4): 543–574.

Aho, Kevin. 2020. "The Uncanny in the Time of Pandemics: Heideggerian Reflections on the Coronavirus." *Gatherings: The Heidegger Circle Annual* 10: 1–19.

Alcoff, Linda Martin. 2008. "How Is Epistemology Political?" In *The Feminist Philosophy Reader*, edited by Alison Bailey and Chris Cuomo. McGraw-Hill.

Altman, Meryl. 2020. *Beauvoir in Time*. Brill.

Altman, Molly R., Monica R. McLemore, Talita Oseguera, Audrey Lyndon, and Linda S. Franck. 2020. "Listening to Women: Recommendations from Women of Color to Improve Experiences in Pregnancy and Birth Care." *Journal of Midwifery & Women's Health*. https://doi.org/10.1111/jmwh.13102.

Anderson, Ellie. 2019. "The Limits of Consent in Sexual Ethics." *APA blog*, April 24, 2019. https://blog.apaonline.org/2019/04/24/women-in-philosophy-the-limits-of-consent-in-sexual-ethics/?fbclid=IwAR028JEerJn2BuPYez5vKr0cm-UImkBkOPiQb5pi0gm4VKGh8X1Z0qm_lz4.

Arp, Kristana. 2001. *The Bonds of Freedom: Simone de Beauvoir's Existentialist Ethics*. Open Court Publishing Company.

Ayers, Susan, Andrew Eagle, and Helen Waring. 2006. "The Effects of Childbirth-Related Post-Traumatic Stress Disorder on Women and Their Relationships: A Qualitative Study." *Psychology, Health and Medicine* 11: 389–398.

Baker, Jen. 2010. "Natural Childbirth Is for the Birds." In *Motherhood—Philosophy for Everyone: The Birth of Wisdom*, edited by Sheila Lintott. Blackwell.

Baker, Sarah R., Precilla Y. L. Choi Carol A. Henshaw, and Joanne Tree. 2005. "'I Felt as Though I'd Been in Jail': Women's Experiences of Maternity Care during Labour, Delivery and the Immediate Postpartum." *Feminism & Psychology* 15 (3): 315–342. https://doi.org/10.1177/0959-353505054718.

Bakhtin, Mikhail. 1965. *Rabelais and His World*. The MIT Press.

Bartky, Sandra Lee. 1990. "Shame and Gender." In *Femininity and Domination: Studies in the Phenomenology of Oppression*. Routledge.

Bauer, Nancy. 2006. "Beauvoir's Heideggerian Ontology." In *The Philosophy of Simone de Beauvoir, Critical Essays*, edited by Margaret E. Simons. Indiana University Press.

Beck, Cheryl Tatano. 2004a. "Birth Trauma: In the Eye of the Beholder." *Nursing Research* 53 (1): 28–35.

Beck, Cheryl Tatano. 2004b. "Post-Traumatic Stress Disorder Due to Childbirth: The Aftermath." *Nursing Research* 53 (4): 216–224.

Beck, Cheryl Tatano, and Sharon Casavant. 2019. "Synthesis of Mixed Research on Posttraumatic Stress Related to Traumatic Birth." *Journal of Obstetric Gynecologic & Neonatal Nursing* 48 (4): 385–397. https://doi.org/10.1016/j.jogn.2019.02.004.

Béhague, Dominique P., Cesar G. Victora, and Fernando C. Barros. 2002. "Consumer Demand for Caesarean Sections in Brazil: Informed Decision Making, Patient Choice, or Social Inequality? A Population Based Birth Cohort Study Linking Ethnographic and Epidemiological Methods." *British Medical Journal* 324 (20): 942–945.

Behruzi, Roxana, Marie Hatem, Lise Goulet, William Fraser, and Chizuru Misago. 2013. "Understanding Childbirth Practices as an Organizational Cultural Phenomenon: A Conceptual Framework." *BMC Pregnancy and Childbirth* 13 (1): 205–214.

Bellhouse, Clare, Meredith Temple-Smith, Shaun Watson, and Jade E. Bilardi. 2018. " 'The Loss Was Traumatic … Some Healthcare Providers Added to That': Women's Experiences of Miscarriage." *Women and Birth* 32 (2): 137–146.

Bellón Sánchez, Silvia. 2014. *Obstetric Violence: Medicalization, Authority Abuse and Sexism within Spanish Obstetric Assistance. A New Name for Old Issues?* MA thesis, Utrecht University.

Bergoffen, Debra. 1997. *The Philosophy of Simone de Beauvoir: Gendered Phenomenologies, Erotic Generosities*. SUNY Press.

Bergoffen, Debra. 2012. *Contesting the Politics of Genocidal Rape: Affirming the Dignity of the Vulnerable Body*. New York: Routledge.

Bodner, Klaus, Franz Wierrani, Werner Grünberger, and Barbara Bodner-Adler. 2011. "Influence of the Mode of Delivery on Maternal and Neonatal Outcomes: A Comparison between Elective Cesarean Section and Planned Vaginal Delivery in a Low-Risk Obstetric Population." *Archives of Gynecology and Obstetrics* 283: 1193–1198.

Bohren, Meghan A., Joshua P. Vogel, Erin C. Hunter, et al. 2015. "The Mistreatment of Women during Childbirth in Health Facilities Globally: A Mixed-Methods Systematic Review." *PLoS Medicine* 12 (6): e1001847.

Bonilla-Escobar, Francisco J., Delia Ortega-Lenis, Johanna C. Rojas-Mirquez, and Christian Ortega-Loubon. 2016. "Panamanian Women's Experience of Vaginal Examination in Labour: A Questionnaire Validation." *Midwifery* 36: 8–13.

Bost, Suzanne. 2005. "Gloria Anzaldúa's Mestiza Pain: Mexican Sacrifice, Chicana Embodiment, and Feminist Politics." *Aztlan: A Journal of Chicano Studies* 30 (2): 5–34.

Bradby, Barbara. 1998. "Like a Video: The Sexualisation of Childbirth in Bolivia." *Reproductive Health Matters* 6 (12): 50–56. https://doi.org/10.1016/S0968-8080(98)90007-6.

Braidotti, Rosi. 1994. *Nomadic Subjects: Embodiment and Sexual Difference in Contemporary Feminist Theory*. Columbia University Press.

Broadmore, Juliet, Michael Carr-Gregg, and J. D. Hutton. 1986. "Vaginal Examinations: Women's Experiences and Preferences." *The New Zealand Medical Journal* 99: 8–10.

Buekens, Pierre. 2001. "Over-Medicalisation of Maternal Care in Developing Countries." In *Safe Motherhood Strategies: A Review of the Evidence*, edited by Vincent De Brouwere and Wim Van Lerberghe. ITG Press.

Butler, Judith. 2004. *Precarious Life: The Power of Mourning and Violence*. Verso.

Butler, Judith. 2009. *Frames of War: When Is Life Grievable?* Verso. Radical Thinkers. Kindle.

Butler, Judith. 2015. *Notes toward a Performative Theory of Assembly*. Harvard University Press.

Butler, Judith. 2016. "Rethinking Vulnerability in Resistance." In *Vulnerability in Resistance*, edited by Judith Butler, Leticia Sabsay, and Zeynep Gambetti. Duke University Press.

Butler, Judith. 2020. *The Force of Non-Violence: An Ethico-Political Bind*. Verso.

Byrne, Veronica, Jonathan Egan, Pádraig Mac Neela, and Kiran Sarma. 2017. "What About Me? The Loss of Self through the Experience of Traumatic Childbirth." *Midwifery* 51 (April): 1–11. https://doi.org/10.1016/j.midw.2017.04.017.

Callaghan, Helen. 2007. "Birth Dirt." In *Exploring the Dirty Side of Women's Health*, edited by Mavis Kirkham. Routledge.

Carel, Havi. 2007. "Can I Be Ill and Happy?" *Philosophia* 35 (2): 95–110.

Carel, Havi. 2016a. *Phenomenology of Illness*. Oxford University Press.

Carel, Havi. 2016b. "Living in the Present: Illness, Phenomenology, and Well-Being." In *The Routledge History of Disease*, edited by Mark Jackson. Routledge.

Carel, Havi, and Ian James Kidd. 2014. "Epistemic Injustice in Healthcare: A Philosophical Analysis." *Medicine, Health Care and Philosophy* 17 (4): 529–540.

Carter, Shannon K. 2009. "Gender Performances during Labor and Birth in the Midwives Model of Care." *Gender Issues* 26 (3): 205–223.

Chadwick, Rachelle. 2009. "Between Bodies, Cultural Scripts and Power: The Reproduction of Birthing Subjectivities in Home-Birth Narratives." *Subjectivity* 27 (1): 109–133.

Chadwick, Rachelle. 2017. "Ambiguous Subjects: Obstetric Violence, Assemblage and South African Birth Narratives." *Feminism & Psychology* 27 (4): 489–509. https://doi.org/10.1177/0959353517692607.

Chadwick, Rachelle. 2019. "Practices of Silencing: Birth, Marginality and Epistemic Violence." In *Childbirth, Vulnerability and Law: Exploring Issues of Violence and Control*, edited by Camilla Pickles and Jonathan Herring. Routledge.

Chadwick, Rachelle, and Don Foster. 2014. "Negotiating Risky Bodies: Childbirth and Constructions of Risk." *Health, Risk & Society* 16 (1): 68–83. https://doi.org/10.1080/13698575.2013.863852.

Charles, Sonya. 2013. "Disempowered Women? The Midwifery Model and Medical Intervention." In *Coming to Life: Philosophies of Pregnancy, Childbirth and Mothering*, edited by Sarah LaChance Adams and Caroline R. Lundquist. Fordham University Press.

Clark, Kristen. 2018. Post on "Birth Monopoly" Facebook page (founded and run by Cristen Pascucci). December 21, 4:53 p.m.

Code, Lorraine. 1991. *What Can She Know? Feminist Theory and the Construction of Knowledge*. Cornell University Press.

Code, Lorraine. 2008. "Taking Subjectivity into Account." In *The Feminist Philosophy Reader*, edited by Alison Bailey and Chris Cuomo. McGraw-Hill.

Cohen, Jeffrey Jerome. 2007. "Monster Culture (Seven Theses)." In *Gothic Horror: A Guide for Students and Readers*, edited by Clive Bloom. Palgrave Macmillan.

Cohen Shabot, Sara. 2008. *On the Grotesque Body: A Philosophical Inquiry on Bakhtin, Merleau-Ponty and Other Thinkers*. Resling. (In Hebrew.)

Cohen Shabot, Sara. 2016. "Making Loud Bodies 'Feminine': A Feminist-Phenomenological Analysis of Obstetric Violence." *Human Studies* 39 (2): 231–247. https://doi.org/10.1007/s10746-015-9369-x.

Cohen Shabot, Sara. 2017a. "Constructing Subjectivity through Labour Pain: A Beauvoirian Analysis." *European Journal of Women's Studies* 24 (2): 128–42. https://doi.org/10.1177/1350506815617792.

Cohen Shabot, Sara. 2017b. "Laboring with Beauvoir: In Search of the Embodied Subject in Childbirth." In *A Companion to Beauvoir*, edited by Nancy Bauer and Laura Hengehold. Blackwell.

Cohen Shabot, Sara. 2018. "Edible Mothers, Edible Others: On Breastfeeding as Ambiguity." In *Rethinking Feminist Phenomenology: Theoretical and Applied Perspectives*, edited by Sara Cohen Shabot and Christinia Landry. Rowman and Littlefield.

Cohen Shabot, Sara. 2019. "'Amigas, Sisters: *We Are Being Gaslighted*': Obstetric Violence and Epistemic Injustice." In *Childbirth, Vulnerability and Law: Exploring Issues of Violence and Control*, edited by Camilla Pickles and Jonathan Herring. Routledge.

Cohen Shabot, Sara. 2020. "Unauthorized Intimate Examinations as/and Sexual Violence: Some Epistemic and Phenomenological Considerations." In *Women's Birthing Bodies and the Law: Unauthorized Intimate Examinations, Power and Vulnerability*, edited by Jonathan Herring and Camilla Pickles. Hart Publishing.

Cohen Shabot, Sara. 2021a. "On Motherhood as Ambiguity and Transcendence: Reevaluating Motherhood through the Beauvoirian Erotic." *Comparative and Continental Philosophy* 13 (3): 207–219. https://doi.org/10.1080/17570638.2021.2002645.

Cohen Shabot, Sara. 2021b. "We Birth with Others: Towards a Beauvoirian Understanding of Obstetric Violence." *European Journal of Women's Studies* 28 (2): 213–228. https://doi.org/1350506820919474.

Cohen Shabot, Sara. 2021c. "Why 'Normal' Feels So Bad: Violence and Vaginal Examinations during Labour—A (Feminist) Phenomenology." *Feminist Theory* 22 (3): 443–463. https://doi.org/1464700120920764.

Cohen Shabot, Sara. 2021d. "'You Are Not Qualified—Leave It to Us': Obstetric Violence as Testimonial Injustice." *Human Studies* 44 (4): 635–653. https://doi.org/10.1007/s10746-021-09596-1.

Cohen Shabot, Sara. 2022a. "Embracing Misfit Bodies: A Reflection on My Brother's Dementia in the Time of COVID-19." *PUNCTA. Journal of Critical Phenomenology* 5 (1): 115–123, Special Issue: Pandemic Politics and Phenomenology. http://journals.oregondigital.org/index.php/pjcp/article/view/4903/5021.

Cohen Shabot, Sara. 2022b. "From Women's Sacrifice to Feminist Sacrifice: Medicalized Birth and 'Natural' Birth versus Woman-Centered Birth." *JRAT—Interdisciplinary Journal for Religion and Transformation in Contemporary Society*, 8: 416–434.

Cohen Shabot, Sara, and Keshet Korem. 2018. "Domesticating Bodies through Shame: Understanding the Role of Shame in Obstetric Violence." *Hypatia* 33 (3): 384–401. https://doi.org/10.1111/hypa.12428.

Cohen Shabot, Sara, and Christinia Landry. 2018. "The Water We Swim In: Why Feminist Phenomenology Today." In *Rethinking Feminist Phenomenology: Theoretical and Applied Perspectives*, edited by Sara Cohen Shabot and Christinia Landry. Rowman and Littlefield.

Cohen Shabot, Sara, and Yaki Menschenfreund. 2008. "Is Existential Authenticity Unethical? De Beauvoir on Ethics, Authenticity and Embodiment." *Philosophy Today* 52 (2): 150–156.

Cohen Shabot, Sara, and Michelle Sadler. 2023. "'My Soul Hurt and I Felt I Was Dying': Obstetric Violence as Torture." *Hypatia*.

Cook, Catherine, and Margaret A. Brunton. 2015. "Pastoral Power and Gynaecological Examinations: A Foucauldian Critique of Clinician Accounts of Patient-Centred Consent." *Sociology of Health & Illness* 37 (4): 545–560. https://doi.org/10.1111/1467-9566.12209.

Creed, Barbara. 1986. "Horror and the Monstrous-Feminine: An Imaginary Abjection." *Screen* 27 (1): 44–71.

Creed, Barbara. 2015. *The Monstrous-Feminine: Film, Feminism, Psychoanalysis*. Routledge.

Creed, Barbara. 2016. "Monstrous-Feminine." In *The Wiley Blackwell Encyclopedia of Gender and Sexuality Studies*, edited by Naples Nancy. Blackwell.

Dahan, Orli. 2019. "Submission, Pain and Pleasure: Considering an Evolutionary Hypothesis Concerning Sexual Masochism." *Psychology of Consciousness: Theory, Research, and Practice* 6 (4): 386. http://doi.org/10.1037/cns0000202.

Dahan, Orli. 2020. "Birthing Consciousness as a Case of Adaptive Altered State of Consciousness Associated with Transient Hypofrontality." *Perspectives on Psychological Science* 15 (3): 794–808.

Dahan, Orli. 2021a. "The Birthing Brain: A Lacuna in Neuroscience." *Brain and Cognition* 150: 1–6. https://doi.org/10.1016/j.bandc.2021.105722.

Dahan, Orli. 2021b. "Obstetrics at Odds with Evolution: The Consequences of Interrupting Adaptive Birthing Consciousness." *New Ideas in Psychology* 63: 100903.

Dahan, Orli. 2021c. "The Riddle of the Extreme Ends of the Birth Experience: Birthing Consciousness and Its Fragility." *Current Psychology* 42 (1): 262–272.

Dahan, Orli. 2023. "Birthing as an Experience of Awe: Birthing Consciousness and Its Long-Term Positive Effects." *Journal of Theoretical and Philosophical Psychology* 43 (1): 16–30.

Dahlen, Hannah, Soo Downe, Margie Duff, and Gill Gyte. 2013. "Vaginal Examination during Normal Labor: Routine Examination or Routine Intervention?" *International Journal of Childbirth* 3 (3): 142–152.

Davis, Dána-Ain. 2019. "Obstetric Racism: The Racial Politics of Pregnancy, Labor, and Birthing." *Medical Anthropology* 38 (7): 560–573. https://doi.org/10.1080/01459740.2018.1549389.

Dawes Gay, Elizabeth. 2018. "Serena Williams Could Insist that Doctors Listen to Her. Most Black Women Can't." *The Nation*, January 18. www.thenation.com/article/serena-williams-could-insist-that-doctors-listen-to-her-most-black-women-cant/.

de Beauvoir, Simone. 1948. *The Ethics of Ambiguity*. Translated by Bernard Frechtman. Philosophical Library. Originally published 1947 as *Pour une morale de l'ambiguïté*. Gallimard.

de Beauvoir, Simone. 2004. "Pyrrhus and Cineas." Translated by Marybeth Timmermann. In *Simone de Beauvoir Philosophical Writings*, edited by Margaret A. Simons. University of Illinois Press. Originally published 1944 as *Pyrrhus et Cinéas*, Gallimard.

de Beauvoir, Simone. 2011. *The Second Sex*. Translated and edited by Constance Borde and Sheila Malovany-Chevallier. Vintage Books. Originally published 1949 as *Le deuxième sexe*, 2 vols. Gallimard.

Dixon-Woods, Mary, Simon J. Williams, Clare J. Jackson, Andrea Akkad, Sara Kenyon, and Marwan Habiba. 2006. "Why Do Women Consent to Surgery, Even When They Do Not Want To? An Interactionist and Bourdieusian Analysis." *Social Science & Medicine* 62 (11): 2742–2753.

Dolezal, Luna. 2015. *The Body and Shame: Phenomenology, Feminism, and the Socially Shaped Body*. Lexington Books.

Douglas, Mary. 1966. *Purity and Danger*. Routledge.

Downe, Soo, Gillian M. L. Gyte, Hannah G. Dahlen, and Mandisa Singata. 2013. "Routine Vaginal Examinations for Assessing Progress of Labour to Improve Outcomes for Women and Babies at Term." *Cochrane Database of Systematic Reviews* 7. Art. No.: CD010088. https://doi.org/10.1002/14651858.CD010088.pub2.

Drouillard, Jill. 2021. "The King Was Pregnant: Reproductive Ethics and Transgender Pregnancy." *IJFAB: International Journal of Feminist Approaches to Bioethics* 14 (1): 120–140.

Edwards, Nadine Pilley. 2005. *Birthing Autonomy: Women's Experiences of Planning Home Births*. Routledge.

Elmir, Rakime, Virginia Schmied, Lesley Wilkes, and Debra Jackson. 2010. "Women's Perceptions and Experiences of a Traumatic Birth: A Metaethnography." *Journal of Advanced Nursing* 66 (10): 2142–2153.

Enkin, Murray, Marc Keirse, James Neilson, et al. 2001. "Effective Care in Pregnancy and Childbirth: A Synopsis." *Birth* 28 (1): 41–51.

Fernández, Ibone Olza. 2013. "PTSD and Obstetric Violence." *Midwifery Today* 105: 48–68.

Ferrazzi, Enrico, Silvano Milani, Federico Cirillo, et al. 2015. "Progression of Cervical Dilatation in Normal Human Labor is Unpredictable." *Acta Obstetricia et Gynecologica Scandinavica* 94 (10): 1136–1144. https://doi.org/10.1111/aogs.12719. Epub Sep. 3.

Fisher, Linda. 2000. "Phenomenology and Feminism: Perspectives on Their Relation." In *Feminist Phenomenology*, edited by Linda Fisher and Lester Embree. Kluwer Academic Publishers.

Flores Ruíz, Elena. 2014. "Musing: Spectral Phenomenologies: Dwelling Poetically in Professional Philosophy." *Hypatia* 29 (1): 196–204. https://doi.org/10.1111/hypa.12066.

Foth, Thomas, and Annette Leibing. 2022. "Rethinking Dementia as a Queer Way of Life and as 'Crip Possibility': A Critique of the Concept of Person in Person-Centredness." *Nursing Philosophy* 23 (1): e12373.

Foucault, Michel. 1979. *Discipline and Punish: The Birth of the Prison*. Vintage.

Foucault, Michel. 2003. *"Society Must Be Defended": Lectures at the Collège de France, 1975–1976* (Vol. 1). Macmillan.

Fricker, Miranda. 2007. *Epistemic Injustice: Power and the Ethics of Knowing*. Oxford University Press.

Garcia, Manon. 2021. *We Are Not Born Submissive*: How Patriarchy Shapes Women's Lives. Princeton University Press.

Garland-Thomson, Rosemarie, ed. 1996. *Freakery: Cultural Spectacles of the Extraordinary Body*. NYU Press.

Garland-Thomson, Rosemarie. 2011. "Misfits: A Feminist Materialist Disability Concept." *Hypatia* 26 (3): 591–609.

Garland-Thomson, Rosemarie. 2020a. "Integrating Disability, Transforming Feminist Theory." *Feminist Theory Reader: Local and Global Perspectives*, edited by Carole McCann, Seung-kyung Kim, and Emek Ergun. Routledge.

Garland-Thomson, Rosemarie. 2020b. "Misfitting." In *50 Concepts for a Critical Phenomenology*, edited by Gail Weiss, Ann V. Murphy, and Gayle Salamon. Northwestern University Press.

Gaskin, Ina May. 2003. *Ina May's Guide to Childbirth*. Bantam Dell.

Gaskin, Ina May. 2011. *Birth Matters: A Midwife's Manifesta*. Seven Stories Press.

Gilligan, Carol. 1982. *In a Different Voice*. Harvard University Press.

Goering, Sara. 2009. "Postnatal Reproductive Autonomy: Promoting Relational Autonomy and Self-Trust in New Parents." *Bioethics* 23 (1): 9–19.

Good, Byron J. 1994. *Medicine, Rationality and Experience: An Anthropological Perspective*. Cambridge University Press.

Gothlin, Eva. 2003. "Reading Simone de Beauvoir with Martin Heidegger." In *The Cambridge Companion to Simone de Beauvoir*, edited by Claudia Card. Cambridge University Press.

Gothlin, Eva. 2006. "Beauvoir and Sartre on Appeal, Desire and Ambiguity." In *The Philosophy of Simone de Beauvoir, Critical Essays*, edited by Margaret A. Simons. Indiana University Press.

Grundström, Hanna, Siw Alehagen, Preben Kjølhede, and Carina Bererö. 2018. "The Double-Edged Experience of Healthcare Encounters among Women with Endometriosis: A Qualitative Study." *Journal of Clinical Nursing* 27 (1–2): 205–211.

Guenther, Lisa. 2020. "Critical Phenomenology." In *50 Concepts for a Critical Phenomenology*, edited by Gail Weiss, Ann V. Murphy, and Gayle Salamon. Northwestern University Press.

Halberstam, Jack. 2011. "The Queer Art of Failure." In *The Queer Art of Failure. A John Hope Franklin Center Book*. Duke University Press.

Halberstam, J. Jack, and Judith Halberstam. 2005. *In a Queer Time and Place: Transgender Bodies, Subcultural Lives*. NYU Press.

Hall, Jenny, Vanora Hundley, Bethan Collins, and Jillian Ireland. 2018. "Dignity and Respect during Pregnancy and Childbirth: A Survey of the Experience of Disabled Women." *BMC Pregnancy and Childbirth* 18 (1): 1–13.

Hall, Kim Q. 2021. "Limping Along: Toward a Crip Phenomenology." *The Journal of Philosophy of Disability* 1: 11–33.

Hall, Priscilla J., Jennifer Whitman Foster, Kathryn M. Yount, and Bonnie Mowinski Jennings. 2018. "Keeping It Together and Falling Apart: Women's Dynamic Experience of Birth." *Midwifery* 58: 130–136.

Harbin, Ami. 2012. "Bodily Disorientation and Moral Change." *Hypatia* 27 (2): 261–280.

Harbin, Ami. 2014. "Disorientation and the Medicalization of Struggle." *IJFAB: International Journal of Feminist Approaches to Bioethics* 7 (1): 99–121.

Harbin, Ami. 2016. *Disorientation and Moral Life*. Oxford University Press.

Harding, Sandra. 2008. "'Strong Objectivity' and Socially Situated Knowledge." In *The Feminist Philosophy Reader*, edited by Alison Bailey and Chris Cuomo. McGraw-Hill.

Harpham, Geoffrey G. 1982. *On the Grotesque: Strategies of Contradiction in Art and Literature*. Princeton University Press.

Harris, Rachel, and Susan Ayers. 2012. "What Makes Labour and Birth Traumatic? A Survey of Intrapartum 'Hotspots.'" *Psychology and Health* 27 (10): 1166–1177. https://doi.org/10.1080/08870446.2011.649755. Epub Jan 31.

Hartsock, Nancy. 1983. "The Feminist Standpoint: Developing the Ground for a Specifically Feminist Historical Materialism." In *Discovering Reality: Feminist Perspectives on Epistemology, Metaphysics, Methodology, and the Philosophy of Science*, edited by Sandra Harding and Merrill Hintikka. D. Reidel.

Hassan, Sahar, Johanne Sundby, Abdullatif Husseini, and Espen Bjertness. 2012. "The Paradox of Vaginal Examination Practice during Normal Childbirth: Palestinian Women's Feelings, Opinions, Knowledge and Experiences." *Reproductive Health* 9 (16): 1–9. https://doi.org/10.1186/1742-4755-9-16.

Hayes-Klein, Hermine. 2014. "Forced Episiotomy: Kelly's Story." *Human Rights in Childbirth*. http://humanrightsinchildbirth.com/kellys-story.

Heidegger, Martin. 1962. *Being and Time*. Translated by John Macquarrie and Edward Robinson. Harper & Row.

Heidegger, Martin. 1993. "What Is Metaphysics?" In *Basic Writings: From Being and Time to The Task of Thinking*, edited and translated by David F. Krell. HarperCollins Publishers.

Heinämaa, Sara. 2003. *Toward a Phenomenology of Sexual Difference: Husserl, Merleau-Ponty, Beauvoir*. Rowman & Littlefield Publishers.

Herring, Jonathan. 2013. *Caring and the Law*. Hart Publishing.

Herring, Jonathan. 2019. "Identifying the Wrong in Obstetric Violence: Lessons From Domestic Abuse." In *Childbirth, Vulnerability and Law: Exploring Issues of Violence and Control*, edited by Camilla Pickles and Jonathan Herring. Routledge.

Herring, Jonathan. 2020. *Law and the Relational Self*. Cambridge University Press.

Hey, Valerie, Catharine Itzin, Lesley Saunders, and Mary Anna Speakman. 1996. *Hidden Loss: Miscarriage and Ectopic Pregnancy*, 2nd ed. Women's Press.

hooks, bell. 1997. "Selling Hot Pussy: Representations of Black Female Sexuality in the Marketplace." In *Writing on the Body: Female Embodiment and Feminist Theory*, edited by Katie Conboy, Nadia Medina, and Sarah Stanbury. Columbia University Press.

Huet, Marie-Hélène. 1993. *Monstrous Imagination*. Harvard University Press.

Humphries, Gretchen. 2001. "You Should Be Grateful." *Birth Matters blog*. www.birthtruth.org/grateful.htm.

Ison, Jess. 2019. "It's Not Just Men and Women: LGBTQIA People and #MeToo." In *#MeToo and the Politics of Social Change*, edited by Bianca Fileborn and Rachel Loney-Howes. Palgrave MacMillan. https://doi.org/10.1007/978-3-030-15213-0_10

Jaggar, Alison M. 1989. "Love and Knowledge: Emotion in Feminist Epistemology." *Inquiry (United Kingdom)* 32 (2): 151–176. https://doi.org/10.1080/00201748908602185.

Jha, Vikram, Zeryab Setna, Aws Al-Hity, Naomi D. Quinton, and Trudie E. Roberts. 2010. "Patient Involvement in Teaching and Assessing Intimate Examination Skills: A Systematic Review." *Medical Education* 44: 347–357.

Johnson, Candace. 2013. "The Political 'Nature' of Pregnancy and Childbirth." In *Coming to Life: Philosophies of Pregnancy, Childbirth and Mothering*, edited by Sarah LaChance Adams and Caroline R. Lundquist. Fordham University Press.

Jordan, Brigitte. 1997. "Authoritative Knowledge and Its Construction." In *Childbirth and Authoritative Knowledge: Cross-Cultural Perspectives*, edited by Robbie Davis-Floyd and Carolyn F. Sargent. University of California Press.

Kafer, Alison. 2013. *Feminist, Queer, Crip*. Indiana University Press.

Karhu, Sanna. 2016. "Judith Butler's Critique of Violence and the Legacy of Monique Wittig." *Hypatia* 31 (4): 827–843. https://doi.org/10.1111/hypa.12271.

Katz Rothman, Barbara. 1982. *In Labour: Women and Power in the Birth Place*. Junction Books.

Katz Rothman, Barbara. 2014. "Pregnancy, Birth and Risk: An Introduction." *Health, Risk & Society* 16 (1): 1–6. https://doi.org/10.1080/13698575.2013.876191.

Kayser, Wolfgang. 1963. *The Grotesque in Art and Literature*. Indiana University Press.

Keltner, Stacy. 2006. "Beauvoir's Idea of Ambiguity." In *The Philosophy of Simone de Beauvoir, Critical Essays*, edited by Margaret E. Simons. Indiana University Press.

Kitzinger, Sheila. 2006. "Birth as Rape: There Must Be an End to 'Just in Case' Obstetrics." *British Journal of Midwifery* 14 (9): 544.

Knowles, Charlotte. 2019. "Beauvoir on Women's Complicity in Their Own Unfreedom." *Hypatia* 34 (2): 242–265.

Knowles, Charlotte. 2021. "Responsibility in Cases of Structural and Personal Complicity: A Phenomenological Analysis." *The Monist* 104 (2): 224–237.

Knowles, Charlotte. 2022. "Beyond Adaptive Preferences: Rethinking Women's Complicity in Their Own Subordination." *European Journal of Philosophy* 30 (4): 1317–1334. https://doi.org/10.1111/ejop.12742.

Kolářová, Kateřina. 2010. Performing the pain: Opening the (crip) body for (queer) pleasures. *Review of Disability Studies: An International Journal*, 6 (3): 44–52.

Kristeva, Julia. 1982. *Powers of Horror*. Columbia University Press.

Kruks, Sonia. 2012. *Simone de Beauvoir and the Politics of Ambiguity. Studies in Feminist Philosophy*. Oxford University Press.

Kuryluk, Ewa. 1987. *Salome and Judas in the Cave of Sex*. Northwestern University Press.

LaChance Adams, Sarah, and Paul Burcher. 2014. "Communal Pushing: Childbirth and Intersubjectivity." In *Feminist Phenomenology and Medicine*, edited by Kristen Zeiler and Lisa Folkmarson Käll. SUNY Press.

Lajoie, Corinne. 2019a. Being at Home: A Feminist Phenomenology of Disorientation in Illness. *Hypatia* 34 (3): 546–569.

Lajoie, Corinne. 2019b. "A Critical Phenomenology of Sickness." *Symposium: Canadian Journal of Continental Philosophy/Revue Canadienne de Philosophie Continentale* 23 (2): 48–66.

Lajoie, Corinne. 2021. "Introduction. Where Goes Critical Phenomenology?" *Chiasmi International* 23: 91–94.

Lajoie, Corinne, and Emily Douglas. 2020. "A Crip Queer Dialogue on Sickness (Editors' Introduction)." *Journal of Critical Phenomenology* 3 (2): 1–14.

Landau, Iddo. 2010. "Violence and Postmodernism: A Conceptual Analysis." *Reason Papers* 32: 67–73.

Langer, Monika. 2003. "Beauvoir and Merleau-Ponty on Ambiguity." In *The Cambridge Companion to Simone de Beauvoir*, edited by Claudia Card. Cambridge University Press.

Leaney, Cindy, and Michelle Silver, dir. 1995. *Unsung Lullabies*. No Time to Cry Productions.

Lebowitz, Leslie, and Jodi Wigren. 2005. "Phenomenology of Rape." *Prepared for the Air Force Sexual Assault Response Coordinator Training Program*, 1–27. www.nationalguard.mil/Portals/31/Documents/J1/SAPR/SARCVATraining/The_Phenomenology_of_Rape.pdf

Leder, Drew. 1998. "A Tale of Two Bodies: The Cartesian Corpse and the Lived Body." In *Body and Flesh: A Philosophical Reader*, edited by Donn Welton. Blackwell.

Letic, Milorad. 2003. "Inaccuracy in Cervical Dilatation Assessment and the Progress of Labour Monitoring." *Medical Hypothesis* 2: 199–201.

Lewin, David, Brenda Fearon, Valerie Hemmings, and Gail Johnson. 2005. "Women's Experiences of Vaginal Examinations in Labor." *Sociology of Health & Illness* 37 (4): 545–560. https://doi.org/10.1111/1467-9566.12209.

Liese, Kylea L., Robbie Davis-Floyd, Karie Stewart, and Melissa Cheyney. 2021. "Obstetric Iatrogenesis in the United States: The Spectrum of Unintentional Harm, Disrespect, Violence, and Abuse." *Anthropology and Medicine* 28 (2): 188–204. https://doi.org/10.1080/13648470.2021.1938510.

Lloyd, G. 1984. *The Man of Reason: "Male" and "Female" in Western Philosophy*. University of Minnesota Press.

Lokaneeta, Jinee. 2016. "Violence." In *The Oxford Handbook of Feminist Theory*, edited by Lisa Disch and Mary Hawkesworth. Oxford University Press.

Loofbourow, Lili. 2018. "The Female Price of Male Pleasure." *The Week*, January 25. http://theweek.com/articles/749978/female-price-male-pleasure.

Lundgren, Ingela. 2011. "The Meaning of Giving Birth from a Long-Term Perspective for Childbearing Women." In *Qualitative Research in Midwifery and Childbirth: Phenomenological Approaches*, edited by Gill Thomson, Fiona Dykes, and Soo Downe. Routledge.

Lyerly, Anne Drapkin. 2006. "Shame, Gender, Birth." *Hypatia* 21 (1): 101–118.

Mackenzie, Catriona, Wendy Rogers, and Susan Dodds. 2014. "Introduction: What Is Vulnerability and Why Does It Matter for Moral Theory?" In *Vulnerability: New Essays in Ethics and Feminist Philosophy*, edited by Catriona Mackenzie, Wendy Rogers, and Susan Dodds. Oxford University Press.

Malacrida, Claudia. 2015. "Always, Already-Medicalized: Women's Prenatal Knowledge and Choice in Two Canadian Contexts." *Current Sociology* 63 (5): 636–651.

Malacrida, Claudia, and Tiffany Boulton. 2012. "Women's Perceptions of Childbirth 'Choices': Competing Discourses of Motherhood, Sexuality, and Selflessness." *Gender & Society* 26 (5): 748–772.

Mardorossian, Carine M. 2014. *Framing the Rape Victim: Gender and Agency Reconsidered.* Rutgers University Press.

Marratto, Scott. 2020. "Intercorporeality." In *50 Concepts for a Critical Phenomenology*, edited by Gail Weiss, Ann V. Murphy, and Gayle Salamon. Northwestern University Press.

Martin, Emily. 1987. *The Woman in the Body: A Cultural Analysis of Reproduction*. Beacon Press.

Martin, Karin A. 2003. "Giving Birth Like a Girl." *Gender and Society* 17 (1): 54–72.

McKinnon, Rachel. 2017. "Allies Behaving Badly: Gaslighting as Epistemic Injustice." In *The Routledge Handbook of Epistemic Injustice*, edited by Ian James Kidd et al. Routledge.

McLeod, Carolyn. 2002. *Self-Trust and Reproductive Autonomy.* MIT Press.

McRuer, Robert. 2006. *Crip Theory: Cultural Signs of Queerness and Disability*. NYU Press.

McWeeny, Jennifer. 2016. "Varieties of Consciousness under Oppression." In *Phenomenology and the Political*, edited by S. West Gurley and Geoff Pfeifer. Rowman and Littlefield.

McWeeny, Jennifer. 2017. "Beauvoir and Merleau-Ponty." In *A Companion to Beauvoir*, edited by Nancy Bauer and Laura Hengehold. Blackwell.

Melo Lopes, Filipa. 2021. "'Half Victim, Half Accomplice': Cat Person and Narcissism." *Ergo: An Open Access Journal of Philosophy* 7 (26): 701–729. https://doi.org/10.3998/ergo.1123.

Merleau-Ponty, Maurice. 1964. *The Primacy of Perception and Other Essays on Phenomenological Psychology, the Philosophy of Art, History and Politics*. Northwestern University Press.

Merleau-Ponty, Maurice. 1968. *The Visible and the Invisible: Followed by Working Notes*. Northwestern University Press.

Merleau-Ponty, Maurice. 1995 [1945]. *Phenomenology of Perception*. Translated by Colin Smith. Routledge.

Miller, Amy Chasteen. 2009. "'Midwife to Myself': Birth Narratives among Women Choosing Unassisted Homebirth." *Sociological Inquiry* 79 (1): 51–74.

Miller, Amy Chasteen. 2012. "On the Margins of the Periphery: Unassisted Childbirth and the Management of Layered Stigma." *Sociological Spectrum* 32 (5): 406–423. https://doi.org/10.1080/02732173.2012.694795.

Miller, Suellen, Edgardo Abalos, Monica Chamillard, et al. 2016. "Beyond Too Little, Too Late and Too Much, Too Soon: A Pathway towards Evidence-Based, Respectful Maternity Care Worldwide." *The Lancet* 388: 2176–2192.

Miller, Suellen, and Andre Lalonde. 2015. "The Global Epidemic of Abuse and Disrespect during Childbirth: History, Evidence, Interventions, and FIGO's Mother-Baby Friendly Birthing Facilities Initiative." *International Journal of Gynecology and Obstetrics* 131: S49–S52. http://doi.org/10.1016/j.ijgo.2015.02.005.

Mingus, Mia. 2011. "Changing the Framework: Disability Justice." *Leaving Evidence* 12.

Murphy, Ann V. 2009. "'Reality Check': Rethinking the Ethics of Vulnerability." In *Theorizing Sexual Violence*, edited by Renée J. Heberle and Victoria Grace. Routledge.

Murphy, Ann V. 2011. "Corporeal Vulnerability and the New Humanism." *Hypatia* 26(3): 575–590. https://doi.org/10.1111/j.1527-2001.2011.01202.x.

Murphy, Ann V. 2012. *Violence and the Philosophical Imaginary*. SUNY Press.

Nirta, Caterina. 2021. "Monstrosity as Resistance: Rethinking Trans Embodiment beyond the Rhetoric of the Wrong Body." *Culture, Theory and Critique* 62: 1–14.

Olza, Ibone, Kerstin Uvnas-Moberg, Anette Ekström-Bergström, et al. 2020. "Birth as a Neuro-Psycho-Social Event: An Integrative Model of Maternal Experiences and Their Relation to Neurohormonal Events during Childbirth." *Plos One* 15 (7): e0230992.

Ortega-Loubon, Christian, Christian López, Franco Romani, and Ricardo Correa. 2009. "Perception and Satisfaction of Users of Public Hospitals in Panama City about Vaginal Examination during Labor." *Revista Peruana de Medicina Experimental y Salud Pública* 13 (2): 1–7.

Pascucci, Cristen, founder. n.d. "Birth Monopoly." Facebook page.

Pérez D'Gregorio, Rogelio. 2010. "Obstetric Violence: A New Term Introduced in Venezuela." *International Journal of Gynecology and Obstetrics* 111: 201–202.

Perrotte, Violette, Arun Chaudhary, Annekathryn Goodman. 2020. " 'At Least Your Baby is Healthy' Obstetric Violence or Disrespect and Abuse in Childbirth Occurrence Worldwide: A Literature Review" *Open Journal of Obstetrics and Gynecology* 10: 1544–1562. https://doi.org/10.4236/ojog.2020.10110139.

Pickles, Camilla. 2015. "Eliminating Abusive 'Care.'" *SA Crime Quarterly* 54: 5. https://doi.org/10.4314/sacq.v54i1.1.

Pickles, Camilla. 2019. "Leaving Women Behind: The Application of Evidence-Based Guidelines, Law, and Obstetric Violence by Omission." In *Childbirth, Vulnerability and Law: Exploring Issues of Violence and Control*, edited by Camilla Pickles and Jonathan Herring. Routledge.

Pickles, Camilla. 2023. "'Obstetric violence,' 'Mistreatment,' and 'Disrespect and Abuse': Reflections on the Politics of Naming Violations during Facility-Based Childbirth." *Hypatia* 38 (3): 628–649.

Pickles, Camilla. 2024. "'Everything Is Obstetric Violence Now': Identifying the Violence in 'Obstetric Violence' to Strengthen Socio-Legal Reform Efforts." *Oxford Journal of Legal Studies* 44 (3): 616–644.

Potter, Joseph E., Elza Berquó, Ignez H. O. Perpétuo, et al. 2001. "Unwanted Caesarean Sections among Public and Private Patients in Brazil: Prospective Study." *British Medical Journal* 323 (17): 1155–1158.

Powers, Jessica, ed. 2009. *Labor Pains and Birth Stories: Essays on Pregnancy, Childbirth, and Becoming a Parent.* Catalyst Book Press.

Ravaldi, Claudia, Miriam Levi, Elena Angeli, et al. 2018. "Stillbirth and Perinatal Care: Are Professionals Trained to Address Parents' Needs?" *Midwifery* 64 (June): 53–59.

Redshaw, Maggie, Reem Malouf, Haiyan Gao, and Ron Gray. 2013. "Women with Disability: The Experience of Maternity Care during Pregnancy, Labour and Birth and the Postnatal Period." *BMC Pregnancy and Childbirth* 13 (1): 1–14.

Reed, Amity. 2008. "Not a Happy Birthday." The F Word: Contemporary UK Feminism, March 7. www.thefword.org.uk/features/2008/03/not_a_happy_bir.

Reed, Rachel. 2011. "Judging Birth." Midwife Thinking, April 9. www.rachelreed.website/blog/assessment-of-labour-progress.

Reed, Rachel. 2015. "Vaginal Examinations: A Symptom of a Cervical-Centric Birth Culture." Midwife Thinking, May 2 (Updated January 2019). https://midwifethinking.com/2015/05/02/vaginal-examinations-a-symptom-of-a-cervix-centric-birth-culture/.

Reeves, Elizabeth A., and Janice C. Humphreys. 2018. "Describing the Healthcare Experiences and Strategies of Women Survivors of Violence." *Journal of Clinical Nursing* 27 (5–6): 1170–1182.
Reynolds, Joel Michael. 2018. "The Extended Body: On Aging, Disability, and Well-Being." *Hastings Center Report* 48: S31–S36.
Reynolds, Joel Michael. 2019. "The Meaning of Ability and Disability." *The Journal of Speculative Philosophy* 33 (3): 434–447.
Reynolds, Joel Michael. 2022. *The Life Worth Living: Disability, Pain, and Morality*. University of Minnesota Press.
Rich, Adrienne. 1986. *Of Woman Born: Motherhood as Experience and Institution*. Norton.
Richland, Shea. 2008. "Birth Rape: Another Midwife's Story." *Midwifery Today* 85 (Spring): 42–43.
Rodriguez-Cayro, Kyli. 2017. "Why Some Members of the LGTB Community Feel Excluded From #MeToo." *Bustle*, October 19. www.bustle.com/p/some-members-of-the-lgbtq-community-feel-excluded-by-the-me-too-hashtag-its-a-reminder-of-how-important-inclusive-language-is-2953162.
Rogers, Wendy. 2014. "Vulnerability and Bioethics." In *Vulnerability: New Essays in Ethics and Feminist Philosophy*, edited by Catriona Mackenzie, Wendy Rogers, and Susan Dodds. Oxford University Press.
Rogers, Wendy, Catriona Mackenzie, and Susan Dodds. 2012. "Why Bioethics Needs a Concept of Vulnerability." *International Journal of Feminist Approaches to Bioethics* 5 (2): 11–38.
Roosevelt, Lee, Megan Diebel, and Ruth E. Zielinski. 2018. "Achieving Competency in Vaginal Examinations: The Challenge of Balancing Student Learning Needs with Best Practice in Maternity Care." *Midwifery* 61: 39–41.
Roupenian, Kate. 2017. "Cat Person." *The New Yorker*, December 11. www.newyorker.com/magazine/2017/12/11/cat-person.
Russo, Mary. 1995. *The Female Grotesque: Risk, Excess, and Modernity*. Routledge.
Sadler, Michelle. 2020. "Despertando las metáforas que dormían en la ciencia (Prólogo)." In *Violencia Obstétrica en América Latina: Conceptualización, experiencias, medición y estrategias*, edited by Patrizia Quattrocchi and Natalia Magnone. Instituto de Salud Colectiva, Colección Cuadernos del ISCo. https://doi.org/10.18294/9789874937506
Sadler, Michelle. 2025. "Obstetric Violence, a Latin American Concept." In *The Routledge Companion to Gender and Reproduction*, edited by Barbara Katz Rothman, Elizabeth Newnham, Rodante van der Waal, and Christie Sillo. Routledge.

Sadler, Michelle, Mário J. D. S. Santos, Dolores Ruiz-Berdún, et al. 2016. "Moving beyond Disrespect and Abuse: Addressing the Structural Dimensions of Obstetric Violence." *Reproductive Health Matters* 24 (47): 47–55. http://doi.org/10.1016/j.rhm.2016.04.002.

Salgado, Heloisa De Oliveira, Denise Yoshie Niy, and Simone Grilo Diniz. 2013. "Groggy and with Tied Hands: The First Contact with the Newborn According to Women That Had an Unwanted C-Section." *Journal of Human Growth and Development* 23 (2): 190–197.

Sandberg, Linn J. 2018. "Dementia and the Gender Trouble? Theorising Dementia, Gendered Subjectivity and Embodiment." *Journal of Aging Studies* 45 (6): 25–31. https://doi.org/10.1016/j.jaging.2018.01.004.

Sandberg, Linn J., and Barbara Marshall. 2017. "Queering Aging Futures." *Societies* 7 (3): 21.

Scarth, Fredrika. 2004. *The Other Within: Ethics, Politics, and the Body in Simone de Beauvoir*. Rowman and Littlefield.

Schalk, Sami. 2017a. Coming to Claim Crip: Disidentification with/in Disability Studies (pp. 123–135). Routledge.

Schalk, Sami. 2017b. Critical Disability Studies as Methodology. *Lateral* 6 (1). https://csalateral.org/issue/6-1/forum-alt-humanities-critical-disability-studies-methodology-schalk/

Schott, Robin May. 2011. "War Rape, Natality and Genocide." *Journal of Genocide Research* 13 (1–2): 5–21.

Shanley, Laura Kaplan. 2012. *Unassisted Childbirth*. Praeger.

Shepherd, Ashley, and Helen Cheyne. 2013. "The Frequency and Reasons for Vaginal Examinations in Labour." *Women and Birth* 26: 49–54.

Shildrick, Margrit. 1996. Posthumanism and the Monstrous Body. *Body & Society* 2 (1): 1–15.

Shildrick, Margrit. 2015. *Leaky Bodies and Boundaries: Feminism, Postmodernism and (Bio)Ethics*. Routledge.

Silva, Michelle Gonçalves da, Michelle Carreira Marcelino, Lívia Shélida Pinheiro Rodrigues, and Rosário Carcaman Toro. 2014. "Obstetric Violence According to Obstetric Nurses." *Revista Da Rede de Enfermagem Do Nordeste* 15 (4): 720–728. https://doi.org/10.15253/2175-6783.2014000400020.

Šimonović, Dubravka (UN Human Rights Council Special Rapporteur on Violence Against Women and Girls, Its Causes and Consequences). 2019. "A Human Rights-Based Approach to Mistreatment and Violence against Women in Reproductive Health Services With a Focus on Childbirth and Obstetric Violence." UN Doc. No. A/74/137. https://digitallibrary.un.org/record/3823698.

Simpson, Madeleine, and Christine Catling. 2015. "Understanding Psychological Traumatic Birth Experiences: A Literature Review." *Women and Birth* 29 (3): 203–207.

Small, Zachary. 2018. "Queer Identity in the MeToo Movement: A Conversation with Emma Sulkowicz." *Hyperallergic*, August 31. https://hyperallergic.com/458257/conversation-with-emma-sulkowicz/

Smeenk, Anke D. J., and Henk A. M. J. ten Have. 2003. "Medicalization and Obstetric Care: An Analysis of Developments in Dutch Midwifery." *Medicine, Health Care and Philosophy* 6 (2): 153–165.

Stawarska, Beata. 2006. "From the Body Proper to Flesh: Merleau-Ponty on Intersubjectivity." In *Feminist Interpretations of Maurice Merleau-Ponty*, edited by Dorothea Olkowski and Gail Weiss. Penn State University Press.

Steele, Alexander. 2023. "The Curious Case of Carson McCullers: Appropriation, Allyship, and the Problem of Speaking for Others." *Disability Studies Quarterly* 42 (3–4).

Steinborn, Maya L., and Emily A. Nusbaum. 2019. "Cripping Human Rights Education with Disability Studies: An Undergraduate Reading List." *Educational Studies* 55 (4): 489–504.

Stewart, Mary. 2005. "'I'm Just Going to Wash You Down': Sanitizing the Vaginal Examination." *Journal of Advanced Nursing* 51: 587–594.

St. Pierre, Joshua. 2015. "Cripping Communication: Speech, Disability, and Exclusion in Liberal Humanist and Posthumanist Discourse." *Communication Theory* 25 (3): 330–348.

Swahnberg, Katarina, Barbro Wijma, and Karin Siwe. 2011. "Strong Discomfort during Vaginal Examination: Why Consider a History of Abuse?" *European Journal of Obstetrics, Gynecology, and Reproductive Biology* 157: 200–205.

Taylor, Dianna. 2018. "Are Women's Lives (Fully) Grievable? Gendered Framing and Sexual Violence." In *New Feminist Perspectives on Embodiment*, edited by Clara Fischer and Luna Dolezal. Palgrave Macmillan.

"They Said to Me." 2021. Facebook page, February 23. www.facebook.com/informedchoicematters.

Thomson, Gill, and Soo Downe. 2008. "Widening the Trauma Discourse: The Link between Childbirth and Experiences of Abuse." *Journal of Psychosomatic Obstetrics and Gynecology* 29 (4): 268–273.

Trigg, Dylan. 2020. "The Uncanny." *The Routledge Handbook of Phenomenology of Emotion*, edited by Thomas Szanto and Hilge Landweer. Routledge.

Tyner, James A. 2023. "The Monstrous-Feminine, the Colonial Body, and Dr. Moreau: Transhumanism, Racial Capitalism, and the Speculative Fiction of Motherless Birth." *Gender, Place & Culture* 30 (9): 1240–1260.

Ussher, Jane M. 2006. *Managing the Monstrous Feminine: Regulating the Reproductive Body*. Routledge.

Vedam, Saraswathi, Kathrin Stoll, Nicholas Rubashkin, et al. 2017. "The Mothers on Respect (MOR) Index: Measuring Quality, Safety, and Human Rights in Childbirth." *SSM—Population Health* 3: 201–210.

Vejlstrup, Jacqueline. 2017. Personal Facebook page. December 28, 10:41 p.m.

Vieira, Tatiana O., Graciete O. Vieira, Elsa Regina J. Giugliani, Carlos M. C. Mendes, Camilla C. Martins, and Luciana R. Silva. 2010. "Determinants of Breastfeeding Initiation within the First Hour of Life in a Brazilian Population: Cross-Sectional Study." *BMC Public Health* 10: 760.

Villarmea, Stella. 2020. "When a Uterus Enters the Room, Reason Goes out the Window." In *Women's Birthing Bodies and the Law: Unauthorized Intimate Examinations, Power and Vulnerability*, edited by Jonathan Herring and Camilla Pickles. Hart Publishing.

Villarmea, Stella. 2021. "Reasoning from the Uterus: Casanova, Women's Agency, and the Philosophy of Birth." *Hypatia* 36 (1): 22–41.

Villarmea, Stella, and Brenda Kelly. 2020. "Barriers to Establishing Shared Decision-Making in Childbirth: Unveiling Epistemic Stereotypes about Women in Labour." *Journal of Evaluation of Clinical Practice* 26: 515–519.

Wagner, Marsden. 2001. "Fish Can't See Water: The Need to Humanize Birth." *International Journal of Gynecology and Obstetrics* 75: S25–S37.

Warner, Michael. 2012. "Queer and Then?" *The Chronicle of Higher Education* 1: 1–7.

Weiss, Gail. 2015. "The Normal, the Natural, and the Normative: A Merleau-Pontian Legacy to Feminist Theory, Critical Race Theory, and Disability Studies." *Continental Philosophy Review* 48 (1): 77–93.

Whisnant, Rebecca. 2017. "Feminist Perspectives on Rape." In *The Stanford Encyclopedia of Philosophy* (Fall), edited by Edward N. Zalta. https://plato.stanford.edu/archives/fall2017/entries/feminism-rape/.

WHO. 2006. *Pregnancy, Childbirth, Postpartum and Newborn Care: A Guide for Essential Practice*. World Health Organization.

WHO. 2018. *WHO Recommendations: Intrapartum Care for a Positive Childbirth Experience*. World Health Organization. Licence: CC BY-NC-SA 3.0 IGO.

Wolf, Allison B. 2013. "Metaphysical Violence and Medicalized Childbirth." *International Journal of Applied Philosophy* 27 (1): 101–111.

Wolf, Jacqueline. 2012. *Deliver Me from Pain. Anesthesia and Birth in America*. Johns Hopkins University Press.

Ying Lai, Chit, and Valerie Levy. 2002. "Hong Kong Chinese Women's Experience of Vaginal Examination in Labour." *Midwifery* 18: 296–303.

Young, Iris Marion. 1980. "Throwing Like a Girl: A Phenomenology of Feminine Body Comportment, Motility, and Spatiality." *Human Studies* 3 (2): 137–156.

Young, Iris Marion. 1997. "Asymmetrical Reciprocity: On Moral Respect, Wonder, and Enlarged Thought." *Constellations* 3 (3): 340–363. https://doi.org/10.1111/j.1467-8675.1997.tb00064.x.

Zigarovich, Jolene. 2018. "The Trans Legacy of Frankenstein." *Science Fiction Studies* 45 (2): 260–272.

Žižek, Slavoj. 2008. *Violence: Six Sideways Reflections*. Picador.

Zorzanelli, Rafaela Teixeira, Francisco Ortega, and Benilton Bezerra Júnior. 2014. "An Overview of the Variations Surrounding the Concept of Medicalization between 1950 and 2010." *Ciência & Saúde Coletiva* 19 (6): 1859.

Index